A Cultural Humility and Social Justice
Approach to Psychotherapy

T0355315

# A Cultural Humility and Social Justice Approach to Psychotherapy

*Seven Applied Guidelines for Evidence-Based Practice*

**ANU ASNAANI**

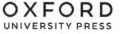

# OXFORD
## UNIVERSITY PRESS

Oxford University Press is a department of the University of Oxford. It furthers
the University's objective of excellence in research, scholarship, and education
by publishing worldwide. Oxford is a registered trade mark of Oxford University
Press in the UK and certain other countries.

Published in the United States of America by Oxford University Press
198 Madison Avenue, New York, NY 10016, United States of America.

Library of Congress Cataloging-in-Publication Data
Names: Asnaani, Anu, author.
Title: A cultural humility and social justice approach to psychotherapy :
seven applied guidelines for evidence-based practice / Anu Asnaani, Ph.D.
Description: New York, NY : Oxford University Press, [2023] |
Includes bibliographical references. |
Identifiers: LCCN 2023003780 (print) | LCCN 2023003781 (ebook) |
ISBN 9780197635971 (paperback) | ISBN 9780197635995 (epub)
Subjects: LCSH: Psychiatry, Transcultural. | Psychotherapy—Cross-cultural studies |
Evidence-based psychiatry—Cross-cultural studies. |
Cultural competence.
Classification: LCC RC455.4.E8 A86 2022 (print) | LCC RC455.4.E8 (ebook) |
DDC 616.89/14—dc23/eng/20230414
LC record available at https://lccn.loc.gov/2023003780
LC ebook record available at https://lccn.loc.gov/2023003781

DOI: 10.1093/oso/9780197635971.001.0001

Printed by Marquis Book Printing, Canada

*To Peter and Neena, who have supported me in more ways
than I can describe, and who show me the beauty and
richness of diversity every day of my life.*

# CONTENTS

The tables, boxes, and exercises provided in *A Cultural Humility and Social Justice Approach to Psychotherapy: Seven Applied Guidelines for Evidence-Based Practice* can also be accessed online by searching for this book's title on the Oxford Academic platform, at academic.oup.com.

**FOREWORD**

In 1989, as a new faculty member in the psychology program at Antioch University, I taught my first course on multicultural practice. I'd come from a doctoral program in clinical psychology at the University of Hawaii, where cross-cultural psychology aligned with transcultural psychiatry and focused on cultures outside the United States. This research was relevant in the broader theoretical sense, but not the kind of practical information my graduate students wanted and needed. In contrast, the beginning field of multicultural counseling focused on people of color in the United States, but with little attention to other marginalized communities or to people of multiple marginalized identities. And unfortunately, the broader field of psychology treated culture as a specialty field irrelevant to the work of psychologists and counselors.

Fast forward to 2023 and it is hard to ignore the topic of culture, especially when it comes to human health and well-being. War, poverty, violence, and natural disasters exacerbated by climate change have contributed to the displacement and migration of millions of people within and across borders. COVID-19 has raised awareness of healthcare disparities in existence long before the pandemic began, and of the ways in which the health of one group affects the entire world. The internet and social media have exacerbated the polarization of people according to political, religious, gender, and racialized identities. And in the United States, hate crimes against people of color, Jews, Muslims, and gay and transgender people have increased in conjunction with overt violence by White supremacy groups.

But approaches to diversity have shifted in some encouraging ways, too. In North America, a growing number of people now marry across ethnic and religious cultures, which has contributed to an increasing number of people who identify as multiracial. Attitudes toward same-sex marriage and gay and transgender people have improved, albeit with a long way to go. Disability culture is gaining visibility, as is the worldwide movement of Indigenous people. Social justice work culminating in the Black Lives Matter and #MeToo movements raised the awareness of many dominant-culture members, with a subsequent growth in DEI (Diversity, Equity, Inclusion) programs in many organizations.

Psychotherapy research, education, and training currently reflect these societal shifts. Thirty years ago, one multicultural class per graduate program was considered sufficient and even progressive in some schools. In contrast, the gold standard of education and training (APA accreditation) now requires infusion of cultural considerations and information throughout coursework, practicum, internship, and post-graduate continuing education. The official definition of evidence-based practice in psychology has expanded from strict experimental designs that left many groups out to "the best available research combined with clinical expertise, in the context of patient characteristics, culture, and preferences."

As a result of these changes, the multicultural clinical/counseling literature has grown enormously. This growth is due largely to an increasing number of psychologists who identify as members of marginalized communities. Approximately 38% of the graduate student population and 34% of early career psychologists now identify as people of color. In addition, an increasing number of psychologists are writing from their personal experience as members of gay, transgender, and nonbinary communities, Disability culture, religions, and other marginalized groups. This increasing diversity of psychologists is occurring in tandem with an increasingly diverse client population.

Dr. Asnaani's book tackles this complexity head-on. She begins with a wealth of personal and professional experience which informs her understanding of the scholarly literature. Her book offers practical information and strategies that therapists will appreciate. And her skill as a teacher comes through in the organization of the book in the form of Guidelines relevant to the practice of psychotherapy. Following each Guideline, she demonstrates its use via a complex case that reflects the real-world identities and challenges facing therapists these days. She weaves four cases throughout the book, along with sections on "Common Challenges" and "Putting It into Practice," ending each chapter with a commentary about how principles of social justice are woven into each topic. She also includes a chapter on the often-neglected topic of relapse prevention and maintenance of treatment gains, and another on the ways to engage in culturally responsive supervision with trainees from diverse identity backgrounds.

Throughout her book, Dr. Asnaani provides examples of nuanced therapist-client interactions in the form of dialogue. This includes helpful information on microaggressions and how to handle them in psychotherapy sessions. Every chapter concludes with a set of excellent discussion questions, with the final discussion question linked to a social justice action.

This well-researched, thoughtfully written book is a very important contribution to the multicultural evolution of psychology. Equally important, it will help therapists of diverse identities and contexts provide the most culturally responsive care possible to a diversity of clients.

Pamela A. Hays, PhD

## REFERENCES

American Psychological Association, Presidential Task Force on Evidence-Based Practice. (2006). Evidence-based practice in psychology. *American Psychologist*, *61*(4), 271–285. https://doi.org/10.1037/0003-066X.61.4.271.

Andoh, E. (2021, April/May). Psychology's urgent need to dismantle racism. *APA Monitor*, 52(3), 38–45.

# Introduction

Before I jump into introducing the topics and motivation for this book, I think it
is helpful to provide a sense of who I am, personally and professionally, and what
perspective I bring because of my own intersectional identities and experiences.
I identify as a woman of color, South Asian in my ethnicity and Saint Lucian as
my nationality, immigrant, cis-gendered, straight, and able-bodied. I trained in
traditional models of cognitive behavioral therapy during my graduate training
at Boston University, specializing in anxiety-related disorders and substance use
disorders, through additional training in the Veterans' Administration system
during practicum and my internship at Brown Alpert Medical School. I have
been fortunate to work with clients, therapists, trainees, and colleagues from a
wide diversity of backgrounds, both nationally and globally, within the contexts
of psychotherapy provision and clinical training in evidence-based approaches.
My research has grown and morphed over time (similar to my cultural awareness and competency as a therapist), originating in traditional experimental
and randomized controlled trial work, and landing squarely on my current preferred interests of community-based research that focuses on addressing health
disparities for a range of diverse communities using a social justice and cross-
cultural lens.

   I think it's important to provide this unfiltered and transparent view of who
I am and what I have learned or taught to others, because, as you will see as we
progress throughout this book, openness, transparency, and willingness to discuss
our own identities (and the strengths and biases they may confer) are crucial to
our quest to become culturally responsive and socially just clinicians. As we weave
our way through the book, I will reflect back on my own biases or gaps in knowledge, and many of the cases we touch on certainly draw from my own missteps
and lessons learned in my own journey. I hope this allows you to be vulnerable
and authentic about your own weaknesses and strengths (and how your identity
and life experiences undoubtedly shape these facets) as you get into the main content of this applied guide.

   Moving on to one of my main motivations for writing this book, one struggle
I often hear from trainees and even seasoned therapists when we talk about the
incorporation of diversity considerations into psychotherapy is that it feels like

*A Cultural Humility and Social Justice Approach to Psychotherapy.* Anu Asnaani, Oxford University Press.
© Oxford University Press 2023. DOI: 10.1093/oso/9780197635971.003.0001

an ambiguous and daunting process to figure out how to do so effectively and consistently. Part of the reason for this lies with the history of research processes in psychology, which proceeded over the past five decades without consideration of how unique identity characteristics of individuals could impact basic (and important) clinical scientific processes from the initial stages of inquiry, leaving us all to play catch-up and figure out the impact of these important factors in a post hoc fashion. Similarly, many of our clinical training models (until the past 5–10 years or so) have pushed for a model of learning about empirically supported or evidence-based treatments as a general model first, followed by modifications based on unique identity characteristics as sort of an advanced or "higher level" standard of training, instead of incorporating such factors early in clinical instruction.

That said, I do want to acknowledge that many brilliant scholars in the field have worked fastidiously and thoughtfully on filling this gap in our focus on the influence of identity characteristics on therapy and clinical practice. Indeed, in creating the current guidelines outlined in this book, I have closely drawn from and referred to a number of published practice guidelines (such as those by the American Psychological Association, 2017, 2019) and the overall body of published literature that have theoretically or empirically examined how best to fuse such diversity considerations into evidence-based clinical practice (many of which I provide as additional resources for readers at the end of this book). Thus, it is important to recognize that when I suggest certain skills to engage in culturally humble practice throughout the chapters of this book, I am generally not making idiosyncratic or personal assumptions about the best way to approach the various identity-related challenges that we experience as therapists. Rather, I am using what culturally competent therapists/clinical researchers have been finding consistently across their work as the basis for my prescriptions. In this way, I am providing what I call "empirically derived" guidelines, so that I can distill the major and repeated points of direction from my esteemed colleagues and expert groups in the field and provide more practical applications of such skills, in order to address the concern that these existing guidelines are either too numerous or difficult to understand in terms of their implementation in a clinical context. If I do make a personal assertion, I will clearly indicate that in the text, as a way of supplementing my teachings with anecdotal suggestions from my own clinical work.

Finally, I want to briefly address one other core element of my work here: the role of *social justice*. As a term that itself is highly related to issues of power and privilege (as we will discuss more as we progress through the book), it is not without its detractors and critics. Historically, the focus on social justice as a necessary movement within our society to address inherent and systematic inequities has belonged to other fields in psychology (e.g., social psychology: Skitka & Crosby, 2003; counseling psychology: Sinacore, Ginsberg, & Kassan, 2013). In clinical psychology, we have often pushed this term aside, believing (in my opinion, erroneously) that it has no place in treatments that are derived from vigorous scientific processes that should work for everyone, regardless of those individuals' own backgrounds or upbringing, and that such a focus would only detract from "active" ingredients that target clinical disorders. It will come as no surprise, given the title of my book, that I do not hold such a belief. In fact, I will make the case throughout this book (drawing on my own research and clinical work and those of a burgeoning number of colleagues in the field) that we have been doing ourselves and certainly those we aim to serve a disservice by not closely integrating a social justice mindset when engaging in evidence-based practice. This will be another theme we come back to repeatedly as we go through this book.

## KEY TERMS

Before I even get into the specific ways we can fuse diversity considerations throughout our clinical practice (from assessment, to case conceptualization, to treatment, and relapse prevention) in each successive guideline, I think it is imperative that we are on the same page about some of the terminology we rely on within this space of good culturally informed clinical practice. This includes some basic, well-established definitions of core concepts (such as diversity and culture), and of concepts that should be (in my opinion) adopted into the mainstream as core concepts because they are highly relevant to the idea of culturally responsive therapy (including concepts such as power, privilege, and social justice). Further, a brief sense of some examples of theoretical models that have guided treatment models in psychology can also be helpful. I briefly cover each of these areas here, and then I conclude this Introduction with a preview of some of the case examples that we will revisit throughout the book to highlight the application of the guidelines that follow.

*Diversity.* Diversity refers broadly to differences humans may show based on any number of identity markers (e.g., race, gender, age, etc.). Recent efforts have included important additions to this term with the use of the descriptors "inclusion" (as a more active integration and explicit celebration of individuals who present with a multitude of identity factors that differ from the default "mainstream" identity) and "equity" (to reflect the growing commitment to equal access, treatment, and opportunities across diverse groups in the field). One exceptionally helpful model that we will refer to often in this book is the ADDRESSING acronym coined by Hays (2022), which is an important shorthand to assist clinicians in recalling the multifaceted (and often concurrent) ways in which individuals can be diverse, and how the concept of diversity extends far beyond one's racial or ethnic identity (which *diversity* as a term has mistakenly become synonymous with). Specifically, this acronym encompasses the identifiers of Age and generational influences, Developmental disabilities, other Disabilities, Religion and spirituality, Ethnic and racial identity, Socioeconomic status/social class, Sexual orientation, Indigenous heritage, National origin, and Gender. Importantly, this model can be applied to clients presenting to a range of evidence-based treatments and the therapists who treat them, thus expanding the ways we think about diversity and identity (and intersectionality) within the context of clinical practice, which contribute to its therapeutic utility.

*Culture.* In my previous writing, colleagues and I have defined culture as a "system of beliefs, perspectives, and values a group of a particular race/ethnicity or geographic region collectively share" (Asnaani & Hofmann, 2012, p. 187). Similar to the idea of diversity, I implore readers to refrain from using *culture* as an interchangeable term for race, ethnicity, or national origin, and to instead think about culture in a more accurate and contemporary use of the term to include other groups which might have shared value or identity systems (e.g., military culture, Deaf culture) (Hays, 2022).

*Cultural competence.* While closely connected to both terms of diversity and culture, particularly within a therapeutic practice context, cultural competence largely refers to the ongoing process of acknowledging and addressing identity differences between the client and the therapist, particularly in terms of the actions of the therapist in this regard (Sue, 1998). Overall, survey data suggest that less than half of therapists actually raise cross-cultural issues with their cross-ethnic/racial clients, and those who do so tend to think that training in cultural competency is important for effective treatment delivery (Maxie & Arnold, 2006). A further feature when considering cultural competency is the two-pronged perception of this ability, i.e., from the client ("How skilled is my therapist in terms of their comfort with raising identity-related issues in session with me?") and therapist perspectives ("How comfortable and skilled am I in raising such issues with my client?"). Per this latter perspective, the Multicultural Orientation Framework (Davis et al., 2018) specifically focuses on elements that have been examined in a research context that refer to the therapist's multicultural competence, as defined by their own cultural humility, assessment of cultural opportunities the therapist identifies within the clinical context to engage in culturally humble practice, and the therapist's cultural comfort in engaging in such exploration of identity facets in therapy.

Notably, the term *cultural competence* is not without controversy. Specifically, training programs and researchers have struggled with how to quantify and measure changes on this construct, and this turns out to be a fairly complicated and not a straightforward process (Tao, Owen, Pace, & Imel, 2015). Further, as I discuss in a bit more detail in Chapter 2 ("Guideline 2: Practicing Cultural Humility as a Continuous Process"), there has been some disagreement around whether the term *cultural competency* or *cultural humility* is more appropriate (Danso, 2018; Greene-Moton & Minkler, 2020). I sometimes use the terms somewhat interchangeably (and I explain why in Chapter 2), though I tend to default to the phrase *cultural humility* to capture this overall concept of improving our skills around working with issues of diversity as they arise in therapy, while maintaining a sense of openness and vulnerability to being wrong about understanding such issues as a therapist, which I think go hand in hand.

*Intersectionality.* As its name implies, this term captures the idea that an individual's various identity markers intersect, interact, and overlap with one another (Nadal et al., 2015). Put more simply, these various factors interact to shape individual experience, worldview, perspective on mental health, and/or interpersonal style with others, which includes particular cultural, national, or racial/ethnic identity characteristics, one's gender identity, age, sexual orientation, and other identity factors, quite similar to the idea proposed by Hays in the ADDRESSING model (Hays, 2022). Much of our clinical practice guidelines have siloed various minority identity groups, which is a simplistic and inaccurate view of how each individual functions as a result of a wider range of identity factors at play (Plaut, 2010).

*Acculturative stress.* Acculturative stress refers to the distress associated with the difficulties that those immigrating may experience due to trying to adjust to the new cultural or societal norms of their new host country (Chou, Asnaani, & Hofmann, 2012; Sirin, Ryce, Gupta, & Rogers-Sirin, 2013). This differs from the idea of acculturation, which is the degree to which individuals coming from a particular cultural context integrate with their new host culture versus continued identification with their original cultural beliefs and practices (Sam & Berry, 2010). Again, this concept can be applied more broadly than just different countries of origin; for instance, conceivably an individual moving from a rural, small-town community to a large urban setting may experience acculturation and acculturative stress processes that will be important to consider within the context of presenting mental health symptoms, given the documented relationship of such processes to mental and physical health outcomes (Sirin et al., 2013).

*Discrimination.* Discrimination has typically been defined as the differential, negative treatment of individuals specifically based on specific identity markers, including race/ethnicity, sexual orientation, gender, disability status, etc. (Asnaani, Majeed, Kaur, & Gutierrez Chavez, 2022). Significant research has been dedicated to the examination of how discrimination is implicated in poorer psychological and physical functioning of individuals from a variety of backgrounds (e.g., Carter, Lau, Johnson, & Kirkinis, 2017; Chou et al., 2012), including the role of discrimination in perpetuating ongoing health disparities in minority identity groups and unequal treatment practices in the health systems (and providers) treating them.

*Microaggressions.* This term is highly related to the concept of discrimination and refers to brief, commonplace insults that are related to one's identity markers. Such insults can be delivered verbally, behaviorally, or via the environment, whether intentionally or subconsciously (Nadal et al., 2015). Similar to other types of discrimination, microaggressions have been implicated in a range of negative mental and physical health outcomes, but their occurrence is even more overlooked or underestimated than overt discrimination (Sue et al., 2007). In fact, significant evidence points to the unfortunately frequent occurrence of microaggressions directed toward individuals who show affiliation with specific minority racial, ethnic, gender, sexual orientation, national origin, and religious groups, and those who identify with a disability. Thus, it is important that we have an awareness and understanding of the microaggressions experienced by those we treat. Of note, therapists in my trainings have occasionally raised the concern that use of the descriptor "micro" somehow diminishes the real and measurable impact that such forms of discrimination have on the well-being of others. As a result, some scholars in the field have preferred use of the term "identity-related aggression" to more accurately capture the impact of such behaviors (see Pinder-Amaker & Wadsworth, 2022). I will generally use the term *microaggression* given its more widespread use at the current time, but I certainly agree with this sentiment that such experiences are in no way less significant or lower in impact because they occur in ways that differ from overt discrimination.

*Power and privilege.* Undoubtedly, our understanding around how societal dynamics and historical injustices to specific minority identity groups have permeated many systems (including healthcare) has grown in recent years. Consequently, it is important to talk about these influences within the context of evidence-based mental health treatment, which has not been immune to the impacts of such forces. Specifically, the concepts of power and privilege are relevant, which refer to the inherent (and historical) benefits for individuals identifying with dominant identity groups that allow them to progress academically, financially, personally, or professionally. These benefits given to dominant identity groups go hand in hand with the concurrent perpetuation of disparities for those not part of these dominant groups by denying minority-identifying individuals these same opportunities based on minority group members' lack of such power or privilege (Knowles, Lowery, Chow, & Unzueta, 2014).

Such explicit exploration of power and privilege within the context of therapy can influence a range of processes occurring within mental health, from access to treatment options, dynamics within the therapy room, to direct impact on the effectiveness of the treatments we deliver, and a recognition of these factors allows therapists who may be coming from dominant-identity backgrounds to unpack their own privilege and serve as more effective allies for reducing disparities for clients coming from minority-identity backgrounds (Knowles et al., 2014). While such concepts have not been systematically integrated into, or tested within, the vast majority of evidence-based treatment protocols we currently utilize in psychotherapy, the growing field of mental health disparities recognizes the urgency in doing so (Asnaani et al., 2022).

*Social justice.* A related term that will be woven throughout the book in our case studies and discussion is social justice. This refers to a growing movement that recognizes the need for mental health providers to use their knowledge and skills to actively advocate for solutions to the persistent health disparities for disadvantaged groups (Horne, Maroney, Nel, Chaparro, & Manalastas, 2019). A growing number of scholars in the mental health field have called for a more concerted effort by psychologists to align their professional pursuits with broader social justice initiatives, such as using effectiveness or efficacy results to directly inform legislation for better mental health reform, or by closely partnering with communities to create a mental health infrastructure that more fully addresses other systemic deficiencies in specific minority or under-resourced groups (Asnaani, Charlery White, & Phillip, 2020). In the context of clinical practice, our guidelines will explore such advocacy efforts alongside the delivery of an evidence-based treatment to guide readers on how to engage in such important efforts from within our clinical roles.

*Evidence-based practice (EBP) and empirically supported treatments (ESTs).* Finally, I want to ensure we are on the same page about what I am referring to as I talk about incorporation of the proposed guidelines into evidence-based practices and treatments. In general, I am referring here to consensus on what constitutes "evidence-based" as delineated by larger therapy governing bodies (such as the American Psychological Association [APA]; e.g., see APA report, 2006) about what treatments have met the standards for rigorous scientific exploration and testing for specific disorders and/or groups of individuals. As a clinical scientist, I rely on the field's pooled knowledge on what treatments seem to work for the majority of people presenting with specific symptoms. That said, I completely understand that many of our EBPs and ESTs have themselves been limited in their inclusion of diverse patient populations when they were developed and tested (La Roche, 2021; Zane, Bernal, & Leong, 2016), and therefore these treatments are not the end-all holy grail for all clients of all backgrounds. However, I still use these treatments as the context for showing application of the proposed guidelines because this is the state of science at the current time, and is in line with what the majority of our trainees and clinicians are being encouraged to utilize. Therefore, I want to provide guidance around how to incorporate diversity considerations and social justice principles while still adhering to what we (currently) know to be the active ingredients of such treatments.

## THEORETICAL MODELS OF IDENTITY FORMATION IN MENTAL HEALTH

As we embark on this quest for cultural competence, I would be remiss to omit at least a brief discussion around some of the important theoretical models underlying identity formation and diversity science more broadly, upon which our clinical practice guidelines have been based. Several of these models are important to consider here; please note that the review here is by no means exhaustive, and a number of scholars in the field have expanded on these frameworks and others (e.g., Quintana, 2007; Sue, Sue, Neville, & Smith, 2022). The first set of models explain how our racial identities develop, whether we identify as a Person of Color (POC) or as White. Cross (1995) delineated one such model for Black racial identity formation, which can certainly be translated to individuals identifying as Black, Indigenous, or People of Color (BIPOC) more broadly, and this is accompanied by a delineation of White racial identity formation as outlined by Helms (1995). Both models are relevant to our understanding of our own racial identities as practitioners and are essential to our own adequate identity self-reflection, a prerequisite for cultural competency (as I cover in more detail in Chapter 1, "Guideline 1: Exploring Your Own Cultural Identity, Beliefs, and Biases Before Providing Therapy").

*POC racial identity formation.* Briefly, the POC racial identity model proposed by Cross describes several distinct stages which POC transition through in the formation of their racial identities (and not always unidirectionally), specifically: (a) *pre-encounter*, which refers to an internalized belief that one's Blackness is deficient, and less desirable, than Whiteness, with an unawareness of the racial implications of such beliefs; (b) *encounter*, when certain events force an individual to acknowledge that racism has a negative impact on their life, and that simply adopting White characteristics will not cause one to be regarded as truly White; (c) *immersion/emersion*, which refers to both wanting to surround oneself with symbols of Blackness or connection with Black peers while simultaneously avoiding symbols of Whiteness; (d) *internalization*, which indicates increasing comfort with one's own racial identity, marked by an openness to exploring and establishing relationships with White individuals who recognize and are respectful of racial differences; and (e) *internalization-commitment*, which marks the final stage of utilizing one's personal sense of Blackness in order to make a commitment to actively addressing and advocating for concerns of Black individuals as a group, while still retaining a strong sense of security around racial identities of oneself and others.

*White racial identity formation.* Similarly important to consider is how individuals identifying as White may develop their own racial identity. The White racial identity model by Helms (1995) therefore similarly outlines six stages of this identity formation: (a) *contact*, where the individual can acknowledge racial differences but does not view any problems with this, and does not necessarily consciously engage in racism toward others; (b) *disintegration*, when one encounters direct evidence that their Whiteness brings with it certain privileges over others, causing the individual to experience shame and guilt, subsequently leading to positive or negative outcomes; (c) *reintegration*, which is when there is a negative outcome of the previous stage, typically with the individual holding an attitude of "blame-the-victim" that's more intense than the contact stage, and which is further characterized by a belief that one may indeed be superior in some way to minority groups (particularly, BIPOC); (d) *pseudo-independence*, which is the first stage of identifying positively with one's race, whereby an individual may approve of efforts to combat racism, but there is a reliance on BIPOC to confront and uncover such acts, with attempts to receive validation from BIPOC that they are not racist; (e) *immersion/ emersion*, which in this model refers to genuine attempts to connect to one's own Whiteness and to other White individuals who are trying to be more actively antiracist; and (f) *autonomy*, which occurs when an individual can simultaneously hold both a positive connection to their Whiteness while also actively engaging in social justice efforts to address racism as an active ally to BIPOC.

I have taken the time here to review the ways in which we can think about racial identity formation for the dominant racial group (White or otherwise, depending on our specific context), because we understand from a social justice perspective that the only way we will actually address health and social disparities is through helping individuals understand their own identities (whether that is in terms of our race, but also more broadly in terms of one's religion, social class, education level, etc.) and how those intersect with those identities that have been historically oppressed. Such reflections are key as we work in a position of power as therapists with our clients.

The second category of theoretical models that I believe is appropriate/relevant to review here is around the impact of identity factors on mental health and stress/health vulnerability for individuals from minoritized/marginalized backgrounds. Again, several such theories exist, but I focus here on the minority stress model (Meyer, 2003), given its popularity and high degree of examination across diverse groups, particularly for individuals identifying as sexual minorities.

*Minority stress model.* The minority stress model generally highlights the discrepancy and conflict that can arise between the differing values of the minority group versus the dominant culture or society, and has been largely conceptualized within the arena of sexual minority identities (Meyer, 2003). Specifically, processes associated with increased psychological stress, such as discrimination/bias toward sexual minorities (e.g., homophobia) or the burdens around having to hide or mask one's sexual identity, interact with one's need to survive and adapt to the particular cultural/societal milieu, thereby increasing the stress experienced by an individual. Meyer (2003) posits that these ongoing stressors from repeated and often lifelong harassment and maltreatment based on one's sexual identity explain the ongoing significant health disparities observed in sexual minority groups (both in terms of higher prevalence of psychological dysfunction, and worse treatment outcomes; Marshal et al., 2011; Rimes, Ion, Wingrove, & Carter, 2019). While conceived specifically for the sexual minority classification, we can certainly envision the extension of this framework to other types of minority stress. Further, understanding the unique interaction of minority stress on overall psychological well-being is an important way to understand how one's own diversity factors interact with the dominant societal identities more broadly, and how this interaction may shape or frame the psychological symptoms that one presents with in therapy.

Importantly, none of these models is meant to exactly capture the individual experience of each unique client we may see, and many other excellent models have been constructed for specific identity groups that I have not covered here (e.g., for those identifying as Hispanic/Latine, Asian American, and biracial, Sue & Sue, 2008; or for those identifying as having a disability, Olkin, 2012). These models are simply ways to guide our conceptualizations of our client beyond their psychopathology, and give us context on those we serve (or our own identity formation!) more broadly. An appreciation for such models can inform our therapeutic strategies, to allow us to more centrally incorporate identity and minority stress aspects when working with our diverse clients.

## IMPORTANCE OF UTILIZING PUBLISHED LITERATURE IN DESCRIBING SKILLS

As we get ready to go into the "meat" of this book, you might notice that I will often return to the idea of ensuring that the guidelines I recommend are well rooted in the published literature and prescribed by scholars in the field, as I mentioned in the beginning of this chapter. As I articulated above, there is a clear reason for why I do this, both in this book and during my in-person trainings. Specifically, as a clinical scientist who greatly values what we bring to the table as practitioners and therapists, I see my job in this book as providing my own clinical wisdom as it overlays with the consensus of my highly knowledgeable colleagues in the field, as evidenced by published literature. Therefore, all guidelines will begin with a (brief) review of the literature that supports them, and will provide references that inform my stated guidelines (arranged by chapter at the end of the book) for readers to further investigate, if they wish. I raise this again here as a reminder that as we progress through the book and build our understanding around how to integrate diversity considerations into specific ESTs and EBPs, that anchoring back to what we know in larger samples, through empirical examination or through more general established practice guidelines, will be key to ensuring we are proceeding with the best practices in mind for an individual client.

## CHAPTER STRUCTURE AND CONTENT

The main seven guidelines for practice are described in the first seven chapters of this book, with one chapter dedicated to each guideline. Each of these guideline chapters will follow a generally similar format: a brief explanation of the guideline, a case application of the guideline in practice, a discussion of the challenges in implementing the recommended guideline, specific ways and suggestions on how to practice the guideline in your current therapy work, and a brief commentary on how social justice principles are interwoven into, and are central to, each guideline. I will end each chapter with some discussion questions, which will include an item for social justice action for you to strongly consider in your own clinical practice.

Chapters will also present specific exercises or figures with additional material to strengthen your practice or understanding of how to build your competency in each individual guideline, and all these worksheets are also in the Appendix, along with a compiled listing of additional readings and other resources that are referenced in each chapter. Chapters 8 and 9 will discuss issues specifically related to how these guidelines can be incorporated into relapse prevention/maintenance of treatment gains and supervision, respectively. Finally, in Chapter 10, I will provide some final thoughts for us to consider practically and philosophically as we take what this otherwise very applied book prescribes out into real-life practice.

## CASE EXAMPLES

As a final precursor to delving into the specific actions we can take to become culturally responsive therapists, it will be essential to understand practical application of the skills we learn in this book. As I mentioned in the chapter content section above, I will therefore sprinkle case examples of how guidelines may be applied or explain why they are recommended to ensure the most effective clinical practice. However, for ease and continuity, I will come back to the four cases delineated below, because of the way these specific cases (who are amalgamations of real cases I have treated or supervised) lend themselves to discussion for multiple guidelines with their rich, intersectional complexity. These case examples will also be helpful to follow throughout the course of their treatment, so that one can see how diversity considerations can be fully integrated over the entire course of specific evidence-based approaches, which I will also describe briefly in each chapter when relevant. So, let's get to know these individuals briefly here, and then we will delve more into each case when they make an appearance in the rest of the book.

## Rohan

Rohan is a 32-year-old Sikh American, straight, cis-gendered male whose parents immigrated to the United States prior to his birth, and they live in a small rural town where there are not many other Sikhs or South Asians in general. He presents with symptoms that appear consistent with a diagnosis of obsessive-compulsive disorder (OCD) and social anxiety. Other stressors of note in his life include some familial pressure to get married within his community and several distinct experiences of racial and religious discrimination. We discuss Rohan in Chapters 1 (on self-reflection on our own identities as therapists) and 4 (on utilizing a variety of sources for treatment planning).

## Massie

Massie is a 46-year-old second-generation Filipinx-American, nonbinary individual who identifies as bisexual, and who has recently divorced after coming out to their family. They present with symptoms that appear to be consistent with major depression and generalized anxiety disorder. They also endorse occasional passive suicidal ideation, but stated they would never consider killing themselves because of a fear of the after-life consequences for doing so, based on their faith. Current stressors are related to the fact that they are currently a single parent of two teenage children, and they identify strongly with their Catholic faith, which causes significant conflict with their sexual orientation. We discuss Massie in Chapters 2 (on practicing cultural humility) and 7 (on identifying and incorporating cultural strengths into treatment).

## Tess

Tess is a 24-year-old Latina, straight, cis-gendered woman who immigrated from El Salvador as a teenager with her mother, and she is currently on DACA status, living in a major U.S. city. She presents to treatment with symptoms that seem most consistent with panic disorder with agoraphobia. Additional stressors include significant tension in her relationship with her mother, who disagrees with Tess's pursuit of higher education in her current graduate degree, and the client's guilt about family left behind in El Salvador. We discuss Tess in Chapters 3 (on assessment) and 8 (on relapse prevention).

## Martino

Martino is a 62-year-old Black, Spanish-English bilingual cis-gendered male (undisclosed sexual orientation) whose family immigrated from the Dominican Republic when he was a child and who was primarily raised in a major city on the East Coast. He is presenting to treatment with symptoms that appear to be consistent with a dual diagnosis of alcohol dependence and post-traumatic stress disorder. He noted that he uses alcohol on a consistent basis to mask distressing memories about several distinct events that occurred during his time serving in the military, two notable ones during his time in the service related to racial discrimination and physical violence perpetrated by his comrades. We discuss Martino in Chapters 5 (on exploring cultural barriers to treatment) and 6 (on addressing discrimination within the context of treatment).

---

These brief descriptions of our four case studies hopefully give us a sense of whom we will be working with as we progress through the skills I describe, and we will learn more about these clients as we return to their individual stories intermittently throughout the rest of this book. Now, let's get started and jump right into "Guideline 1: Exploring Your Own Cultural Identity, Beliefs, and Biases Before Providing Therapy".

# 1

# Guideline 1

## *Exploring Your Own Cultural Identity, Beliefs, and Biases Before Providing Therapy*

### GUIDELINE 1 EXPLAINED

As we focus on our desire to be culturally competent and responsive in our provision of evidence-based practices (EBPs) with clients of many different identities, the first step is actually to focus on understanding the impact of our own intersectional identities on the therapy dynamic (Plummer, 1997). Further, it is important to consider (as we reviewed in the Introduction) that the concept of "cultural competence" is not just a therapist's understanding of their own ability to navigate or address diversity or identity-related issues in therapy, but also the client's perception of the therapist's cultural competence (Maxie & Arnold, 2006; Owen, Leach, Wampold, & Rodolfa, 2010). A client's perception of their therapist's cultural competence can certainly be influenced by (1) the therapist's own reflection on how their identity may influence the alliance, and (2) the therapist's own relational dynamic with clients of different backgrounds (whether a racial/ethnic, socioeconomic, sexual orientation, gender identity, religious, or any number of diversity-marker differences that are apparent between therapist and client).

Let's pause here so that we can start this self-reflection process (which is a profession-long pursuit which will likely morph and progress over time). Still, take a few minutes to reflect on where you stand currently on the following as outlined in Exercise 1.1 (all worksheets can also be found in the Appendix).

*A Cultural Humility and Social Justice Approach to Psychotherapy.* Anu Asnaani, Oxford University Press.
© Oxford University Press 2023. DOI: 10.1093/oso/9780197635971.003.0002

Exercise 1.1

## Self-Identification Worksheet

| Identity Factor | How Others Identify Me | How I Identify |
|---|---|---|
| <u>A</u>ge and generational influences | | |
| <u>D</u>evelopmental disabilities | | |
| <u>D</u>isabilities (other) | | |
| <u>R</u>eligion and spirituality | | |
| <u>E</u>thnic and racial identity | | |
| <u>S</u>ocioeconomic status/social class | | |
| <u>S</u>exual orientation | | |
| <u>I</u>ndigenous heritage | | |
| <u>N</u>ational origin | | |
| <u>G</u>ender | | |

(Based on ADDRESSING model; Hays, 2022)

**What Do I Struggle with about My Own and Others' Diversity Markers in Society?**

In addition, cultural competence is not achieved simply by identifying or naming cultural/identity differences between the therapist and client (Sue & Zane, 2009). Instead, experts in the field offer that it is valuable to make the effort to engage in a self-reflection that includes an authentic and honest examination of one's own community-based/personal attitudes toward mental health and treatment-seeking (e.g., Chung & Lu, 1996) and to acknowledge one's own biases toward specific diverse groups (e.g., toward members of the queer community; Carvalho et al., 2022). Related to this self-reflection, therapists are empowered to discuss the issues that arise from such introspective work with their professional peers and supervisors in order to address any potentially cross-cultural conflicts that may impede the working alliance during the course of an EBP (Asnaani & Hofmann, 2012). Such effortful reflection and explicit discussion show an appreciation for the bidirectional influence of identity factors in therapy, and are conceptualized as facilitating a healthy and effective dialogue about sensitive cross-cultural topics that might arise in the context of treatment.

Exercise 1.2 provides a structure for how to engage in such additional self-reflection on one's own biases and internalized stigma, and ways to address such biases in order to provide the best level of clinical care to one's clients.

Exercise 1.2

## Self-Reflection on Biases and Internalized Stigmas

1. **Ask** yourself:
   a. What negative judgments have I noticed I make about others based on their race, gender, sexual orientation, religion, or any number of identity factors?

   b. What negative judgments have others made about my own identity characteristics? Which of these have I also had about myself or others who identify similarly?

   c. How do I feel about psychological therapy and how useful it would be for me personally if I were struggling with a mental health problem, or if someone in my family were struggling? Would I be embarrassed to receive therapy or have a close family member receive therapy?

2. **Try** an implicit association test that tries to assess your implicit, unconscious biases based on race, gender, stigma toward treatment, and so on. Doing such tests will allow you to access the quick negative judgments we might make about others based on identity factors, including biases and internalized stigma we may not even be aware that we have as mental health providers (Hall et al., 2015). Check out a range of such tests offered via Project Implicit: https://implicit.harvard.edu/implicit/selectat est.html.

   NOTE: This is simply to provide some additional information about your biases and should not be solely relied on as the only assessment of one's own biases.

3. **Engage** your peers and supervisors in an open, honest discussion about these observed internal biases or feelings of stigma toward therapy as a whole. A tip: Mention your own observations or struggles and encourage others to do the same so it feels less alienating or that the problem only lies in your own beliefs (most of us have biases, it's a part of human nature!). If you're a supervisor, share your own to encourage your trainees to do the same.

4. **Strategize** how you can overcome these biases, including being mindful of stigmatizing or negative thoughts during therapy with certain clients (or supervisors or supervisees), raising them in supervision or with close colleagues, or seeking your own therapy to better understand why these biases exist and how to address them so they do not impede the quality of care you provide.

Undoubtedly, such self-reflection about our own identification and internal biases is likely beneficial to our ability to feel and appear more culturally competent when providing therapy. The question that remains is, how do we extend past a self-reflection and some basic action skills related to such a reflection, as prescribed in Exercises 1.1 and 1.2, to grow and improve as clinicians for clients of all identities? Even more importantly, perhaps, how do we fuse this effort with our knowledge of effective treatment in the therapy room? Take the example of the situation that arose in case review and supervision prior to the therapist starting to work with one of our cases, Rohan, who differed on a number of diversity factors from the therapist and the supervisor.

## CASE APPLICATION

*Case description.* Rohan is a 32-year-old Sikh American, straight, cis-gendered male whose parents immigrated to the United States prior to his birth; they live in a smaller, rural town where there are not many other Sikhs or South Asians in general. He has completed his bachelor's degree in Business Studies and now assists in running the family business with his parents. He presents with symptoms that appear consistent with a diagnosis of obsessive-compulsive disorder (OCD), including significant rituals (compulsions) related to his personal grooming (some of which connect to religious practices in maintaining his facial hair and ensuring tidiness of his turban) that also extend to some general cleanliness compulsions (excessive hand-washing, showering, and cleaning of house surfaces). In addition, Rohan reports feeling very socially anxious ("self-conscious") when around others not in his direct family or friends circle, including new customers who come to the store, meeting new people at the temple, and when being in public in general, with a fear that he looks odd or might make others uncomfortable with his presence. Other stressors of note in his life include some familial pressure to get married (ideally to someone from the Sikh community) and several distinct experiences of racial and religious discrimination based on beliefs that he is Muslim, including one incident where he was spat on and called a racial slur when waiting in line for a concert with friends.

*Evidence-based treatment approach.* Based on the client's chief complaints of cleanliness compulsions and accompanying distress related to thoughts of contamination, the chosen EBP is exposure and response prevention (E/RP; Foa, Yadin, & Lichner, 2012), a front-line treatment for OCD. Briefly, this approach includes engaging clients in gradual approach of feared situations, thoughts, and objects that may bring on obsessions or avoidance responses that are typical in OCD, with in vivo and imaginal exposure activities being key components within this approach. Treatment typically occurs once to twice a week for 60–90-minute sessions, with anywhere from 10 to 20 sessions considered to be a full "course" of E/RP.

*Preamble to therapy dialogue.* The therapist treating Rohan was a 24-year-old, straight, White (of Irish descent), cis-gendered female, who was about to start providing therapy to Rohan as part of her third-year practicum within the context of her clinical psychology graduate degree. The therapist was assigned to his case because she had both an open slot in her practice caseload, and she expressed a desire to have cases with primary OCD to gain more practice in her implementation of E/RP. As she reviewed the case prior to her supervision meeting with her supervisor, who was a 43-year-old, straight, Latina cis-gendered female, the therapist was aware of several key thoughts that came up as she reviewed the case: (1) "This client presents with personal grooming compulsions; is this normal for OCD?"; (2) "What do Sikhs believe in and are some of his compulsions normative in that faith?"; and (3) in terms of his social anxiety, Rohan identifies as Sikh and wears a turban, therefore "is it unreasonable for him to be concerned about others judging him or making assumptions about his faith if they are unfamiliar with his religious or cultural practices?"

The therapist decided to bring these and other thoughts she was aware of as she started conceptualizing treatment for this case to supervision. In the following dialogue between the therapist and her supervisor, the supervisor tries to create a space for the therapist to share these reflections and guides her through a more thorough self-reflection as prescribed in this chapter in preparation for meeting with Rohan.

**Therapist**: *So, one of the things I am a bit confused about in terms of how to proceed with this case is the fact that the client raised his Sikh faith as being both important to him but also related to his grooming compulsions during his intake. I am a bit unclear on how excessive his grooming behaviors are since I'm not very familiar with this faith, and I feel uncertain about how to ask him about it (and about his faith in general) without offending him.*

**Supervisor**: *Those are both very fair concerns, and I'm glad you're bringing up your uncertainty here so we can explore it to figure out the most helpful way to proceed. Before we get into those two major concerns, I'd like to ask you if you can reflect a bit on what your own identity markers are (across the spectrum of gender, race, religion, and so on) and how this may intersect with this client's own identity markers in general. What are the likely areas of your respective identities where your and his life perspectives may be most different? Where might they be similar?*

**Therapist**: *Well, the most salient parts where we may differ might be that I identify as female and him as a male, I identify as White and mainstream American culture, and he identifies as . . . well, I don't know if he identifies as Asian or as just Sikh. That's one other thing I'm unclear on. And of course, he identifies as Sikh, and I grew up Catholic but I'm more or less atheist. We may be similar in terms of our education level—I read he got his Master's degree— and he grew up here I believe, so he will likely have some of the same cultural beliefs or societal perspectives. We're also not too far apart in age.*

**Supervisor**: *Great. Now, let me ask you a bit harder question: how are you both similar or different in terms of the privilege you hold based on your salient identity markers, like being White, and the power dynamic in the room, given you are the therapist and he is the client?*

**Therapist**: *Hmmm. That one is a bit trickier—on the one hand, I get that I have more privilege as a White person, and he has on the intake reported being discriminated against because of his religious attire and probably because of his skin color. On the other hand, as a woman, I am often sidelined or underestimated, and I wonder if he also might think I'm less of an authority figure and have less power in the therapy relationship in his culture if men tend to dominate in his community—I am not sure about this, but that might be a guess.*

**Supervisor**: *Interesting, and thanks for sharing some of your own preconceptions of how he may or may not regard you based on your gender. That leads me to another tough question: what biases or beliefs are you finding swirling in your mind when you review this case? I hear one of them is that he may not value you and your expertise as much if his culture is more patriarchal, is that right? What else are you aware of that you think about him or about what he's presenting with, if you're being completely honest? There is no judgment here, but I want us to fully explore how you feel about this case before we dive in to devising treatment or figuring out how to approach him to answer some of our questions.*

**Therapist**: *Well, yeah, I worry he won't take me as seriously if men tend to be the decision-makers in his community as I know is the case for some Asian cultures. Also, I think I feel uncomfortable with just not really knowing what it means to be Sikh—what do individuals from this faith believe? Why do they wear turbans? How does this practice relate to OCD? I feel very uncertain.*

**Supervisor**: *That is all very reasonable to be uncertain about. I certainly have some uncertainty myself about what his faith entails. I know one bias of my own that I was aware that came up for me was that I often find it hard to understand the difference between someone who is wearing a turban because they are Sikh from someone who is part of the Taliban, which strikes a bit of anxiety and even fear in me because of the associations I have with the Taliban. This certainly even brings up some shame for me to say out loud, but I know it's important to share some of the biases and personal emotions I have that come up around this client, because I don't want to hide these feelings and risk providing sub-standard supervision about this client. Do you feel similarly or have other feelings/thoughts that may feel particularly difficult to raise out loud?*

**Therapist** [sheepishly]: *Yes.* [Sighs]. *I hate to say it out loud, but I can tell I am finding it hard to empathize with the client's reports about being discriminated against because he is mistaken for a terrorist, because part of me is . . .* [takes deep breath]*saying, like, well, you do look like a terrorist. Am I just horrible for thinking this? No one should be mistreated for how they look or their faith. And that's also part of my confusion about his social anxiety symptoms—he is worried he will look weird or odd to others, but is this concern actually justified given it might bring up such feelings in others who are unfamiliar with his faith and why he wears a turban?*

**Supervisor**: *I'm so proud of you for bringing up all of these difficult, and I know, shameful sort of thoughts given we pride ourselves as therapists who are objective and here to help all of our clients. And yet, it is SO important that you own and then explicitly raise the very biases that arise for you, particularly as they directly relate to the empathy you want to have for this client, and therefore can directly impact our treatment of his OCD and social anxiety. In making these biases explicit and putting them on the table, we can actually have a chance to work through them and be the type of therapist you want to be, one who is a supportive and therapeutic agent for change for all the clients we see and care for. Let's start to explore how we can address these biases (for both of us), and I also encourage you to continue to be mindful of how these thoughts pop up when interacting with your client, and bringing those observations here to supervision for us to discuss, along with the specific therapy strategies we are going to use to address his symptoms, okay?*

**Therapist**: *Thank you, and I will. That was really difficult to say out loud, but I'm glad we can talk about those things here. I really do want to learn more about his faith and him as a person, and become more comfortable with exploring and addressing such biased thoughts, to be as helpful to him as I can. Thank you for letting me raise those issues here in supervision.*

*Summary of guideline application.* Thus, as exemplified by this exchange, the supervisor encourages the therapist to engage in the self-reflection prescribed by Guideline 1. Specifically, she charges the therapist to think about (1) her own identity markers and how they are similar to or different from the client's stated or salient identity markers; (2) how issues of power and privilege may be at play, and as the case study shows, there is not a clear-cut assessment of these two constructs here as several intersectional identity factors (gender vs. cultural background) are at play; and (3) what biases or discriminatory thoughts the therapist might have toward the client. Importantly, the supervisor models vulnerability and cultural humility (which we discuss in more detail in Chapter 2) by describing some of her own observed biases and areas where she is less culturally informed, to actively create a safe space for the therapist to raise her own similar thoughts. Further, the supervisor provides the rationale for sharing such difficult (and sometimes shameful or embarrassing) beliefs explicitly in supervision, highlighting that doing so provides both the supervisor and therapist a chance to address these biases in order to optimize best treatment practices for the client (which we explore how to do in more detail in upcoming chapters).

## COMMON CHALLENGES

As with any of the guidelines we discuss in this book, there are clear challenges to implementation of Guideline 1 (see Box 1.1). It is my hope that by being aware of the challenges herein, you will be more equipped to address them, both by referring to the Case Application that provides some direction on practical ways to do so, along with the practice tips in the next subsection.

Box 1.1

COMMON CHALLENGES IN IMPLEMENTING GUIDELINE 1

* Therapist denial or lack of awareness of inherent biases based on others' identity factors
* Therapist shame around biases that one is aware of, or shame/discomfort about the salience of one's own identity markers to others
* Anger around having to address one's identity markers within professional settings due to personal history of discrimination or conflict around these identity markers
* Lack of support institutionally or in one's training to explore one's identity factors (e.g., devaluing of such a process by supervisors, trainers, or administrators)
* Uncertainty about how to engage in such a reflection in order to improve cultural competence (tip: check out Exercises 1.1 and 1.2 in this chapter).

First, it is highly possible that we may deny or be unaware of our own inherent biases toward others; this is a normal, expected occurrence, as we are socialized as therapists to regard ourselves as caretakers and sources of support to others by our very profession. That said, this inability to recognize and own our gaps in knowledge about our patients' identities is a potentially dangerous one, which may threaten our ability to be effective, impartial, and to build a strong alliance toward achieving common goals with our patients (Asnaani & Hofmann, 2012). It is possible that our own shame or discomfort around having biases, or even about our own salient identity factors and how those are received by our clients, influences our ability to recognize and verbalize our biases (toward ourselves or others). We explore the concept of cultural humility in Chapter 2, which provides a way to practice owning missteps and biases until such a practice becomes second nature.

However, it's also important to consider that addressing the discrepancy between one's identity markers as a therapist and those of our clients (or even our supervisors) can bring up other emotions, such as anger or frustration, given therapists' own personal history of discrimination or identity-related conflict in professional contexts (e.g., Kelly & Greene, 2010). Often, this frustration is compounded by a lack of institutional support, or little attention paid toward exploring the impact of one's own identity during one's training, a deficiency that many of our psychology training programs have been more actively targeting in the past decade (Mangione, Borden, Nadkarni, Evarts, & Hyde, 2018). Supervisors, instructors, and trainers using this book as a way to guide this process, particularly in trainees from diverse backgrounds, are particularly advised to be aware of other contextual factors that could impede a trainee from being willing or able to discuss cultural gaps in knowledge (see Chapter 9 for more on incorporating the guidelines into the clinical supervision context).

Finally, one of the biggest barriers that stop us from engaging in any new behavior is the uncertainty on how to do so—lucky for you, this chapter itself provides several ways to practice the "how" and address this barrier, from doing the prescribed exercises, reading the Case Application, and reminding yourself of the other specific ways to practice what you have learned here in the next section.

## PUTTING IT INTO PRACTICE

So, at this point, you hopefully understand why we should care about in-depth and authentic self-reflection about our own biases, cultural identities, and relationship to power and privilege in therapy. You also have a sense of how this plays out practically in the clinical setup with clients, and what roadblocks might present themselves to engaging in such crucial self-reflection. Now, as with every good skill, we need to practice. And practice. And practice some more, and do so **continuously** throughout our careers. This is not a milestone that we can check off or be completely actualized in; similar to the idea in values-based therapies (e.g., Roemer & Orsillo, 2020; Zhang et al., 2018), we must treat such self-exploration and reflection as a direction we keep moving in as clinicians, instead of a finite, concrete goal or destination that is reached (see Box 1.2).

The first way to practically engage in this practice is to refer back to Exercise 1.1 in this chapter, followed by Exercise 1.2. The salience of our own identity factors, as outlined in Exercise 1.1, change over time and over the course of our experience as clinicians and academics; similarly, our biases, prejudices, and power-privilege status also morph over time. Thus, these exercises should be part of a self-competency upkeep and evaluation that we do for ourselves on a regular basis, ideally every year or in every new practice setting (whichever comes first), so that we are continuously honing this ability and ensuring we do not generate

---

Box 1.2

### How Do I Practice Guideline 1?

1. **Engage** in Exercises 1.1 and 1.2 (sequentially) as a baseline step; **repeat** every year or in every new practice setting/training level to assess changes to your own identification and assessment of internal biases.
2. **Advocate** for regular programming on cultural reflection/competency/ power/privilege issues in your program, clinic, or local organization of practitioners to keep this skill sharp.
3. **Join** a local or national organization that prioritizes cultural competency efforts or already has a trove of archived programming in this area, and **commit** to incorporating review of such material in your yearly self-upkeep and continuing education as a clinician.

---

any cultural gaps in knowledge that threaten the quality of our culturally responsive care.

Another helpful practice tip is to raise the possibility of a structured, program-wide or clinic-wide investment into inviting continuing education speakers and trainers in cultural competency who can raise issues related to our own privilege and identities in the clinical domain. For those in private-practice settings, this could mean appealing to your local practitioners' organization or state board to ensure such programming is offered regularly, so we all get a chance to continue to sharpen this skill, as it inevitably becomes duller over time and years in the same practice setting. If inviting speakers to some formalized training series within your practice, program, or clinic is not possible, it is incumbent upon each of us (from a social equity and social justice perspective) to join professional practice divisions (e.g., one of the many that are part of the American Psychological Association or any other number of national general or specific practice-oriented organizations) that offer such regular programming or have archives of such trainings that we can partake in on an annual basis (if not more often). Given the distinct and ongoing health disparities persisting for many minoritized communities we serve, particularly around experiences of discriminatory service provision that many such individuals still endure (Hall et al., 2015), it is our responsibility to ensure that we are consistently engaging in our own reflection to bring the most unbiased, equitable clinical practice to every one of our clients.

## COMMENTARY ON INCORPORATING SOCIAL JUSTICE

This chapter is imbued with ways to practice social justice within the implementation of this guideline (as discussed in the immediately preceding paragraph on ways to practice this guideline and as exemplified in the discussion of the ways we can most equitably approach differences between the therapist and our case study, Rohan). Indeed, when we take the time as therapists to better connect with our own strengths and limitations based on our own upbringing and intersectional identities, we are already engaging in more socially just clinical practice. If I lack insight into my own profiles of privilege and power, how can I be certain that I will engage in equitable and non-discriminatory treatment provision? Put more positively, the very (often difficult) effort to do our own self-reflection and assessment (instead of the dominating view in much of clinical psychology that prioritizes focus on the conceptualization of the client only) is a way to directly and individually target health disparities in mental health delivery impacting clients coming from a range of minoritized backgrounds. Do not underestimate the power of authentic and honest self-reflection as a therapist when you find yourself asking the question, "How can I, in my limited range of professional activity, possibly address the persisting inequality in mental health?" Consciously and consistently practicing this guideline is a step in doing just that.

## DISCUSSION QUESTIONS

1. What are the advantages and disadvantages of broadening one's scope of identity focus on factors that extend beyond race and ethnicity? What do you think about the idea that everyone has a diverse, unique identity?
2. How do you think this process of therapist self-reflection differs between therapists from more or less saliently minoritized backgrounds? How about with more or less saliently minoritized supervisors?
3. What barriers or challenges to implementation of this guideline have we not considered that may be unique to your current practice or training setting?
4. What are some potential solutions to these specific complicating factors? How can we apply the basic principles underlying this guideline to the unique barriers at hand in your practice or training setting?
5. **Social Justice Action**: What suggestions do you have for ensuring that such an identity reflection and discussion around internalized stigma and biases are more systematically addressed in our practice or academic institutions? This could be thinking about ways to incorporate such exercises or discussions at an institutional, programmatic, clinical competency, or curricula level within your current work domain.

# 2

# Guideline 2

## *Practicing Cultural Humility as a Continuous Process*

## GUIDELINE 2 EXPLAINED

In my previous culturally competent clinical trainings, I often referred to this idea of cultural humility as an afterword concept in which to think about application of the other guidelines I provide. As my own cultural competence and knowledge have grown, I have realized that the apt place to talk about cultural competency indeed lies at the *beginning* of our pursuit to provide culturally responsive evidence-based treatment, and it should set the frame for all the work we endeavor to do as mental health professionals in this regard. Thus, our second guideline serves as an early reminder of the importance of taking a culturally humble approach to our work as therapists and clinical supervisors, and we will refer back to it throughout the remaining guidelines.

So, what is cultural humility? Cultural humility refers to the process of continuing to be humble about one's knowledge about the impact of cultural factors in psychology and on the therapeutic dynamic (Vasquez & Johnson, 2022), with the understanding that this is a career-long process (Foronda, Baptiste, Reinholdt, & Ousman, 2016). Further, this skill calls for an openness and curiosity by the therapist about how their client views the world, along with a suspension of one's own ego and considerable self-reflection about one's own biases, and conflicting worldviews with a client (Hook, Davis, Owen, Worthington, & Utsey, 2013; Owen et al., 2016). The Multicultural Orientation Framework (Davis et al., 2018) helpfully expands on how we can instead conceptualize cultural competence as consisting of one's cultural humility, and how this is supported by the other two main pillars of this framework, namely the therapist's willingness to make use of cultural opportunities in therapy to explore the influence of identity facets on the target areas, and the therapist's comfort before, during, and after such exploration. Other scholars in the field have further encouraged clinicians to operate from a critical consciousness standpoint in order to engage in such culturally humble processes, which includes being critical of one's ability to be open/

*A Cultural Humility and Social Justice Approach to Psychotherapy.* Anu Asnaani, Oxford University Press.
© Oxford University Press 2023. DOI: 10.1093/oso/9780197635971.003.0003

ego-less, of one's motivations and level of self-awareness, and of one's actions in order to be actively culturally humble (Lee & Haskins, 2021).

However, as reasonable as this sounds (at least to me!), cultural humility is not a concept without controversy, largely stemming from disagreement as to the way it is termed and whether it should be interchangeable with the concept of cultural competence (for some great commentaries and historical perspectives on the debate in various related healthcare fields, look at Danso [2018] and Greene-Moton & Minkler [2020]). In addition, I have heard individuals in my trainings express concern about the perceived passivity of such a crucial skill in the diversity, equity, and inclusion space, arguing that simply being humble and owning up to one's cultural missteps is no longer sufficient given long-standing inequities and maltreatment of various minority-identity groups. While I certainly appreciate and understand this perspective, the idea of cultural humility as it is currently defined appeals to me as a mental health provider because it's largely related to my own professional values of approaching situations as a novice and being open to learning and growth, throughout one's career, regardless of years of experience in the field.

This core component of lifelong learning in the concept of cultural humility has been highlighted by scholars in the field, who note that cultural humility can be garnered throughout the entire expanse of one's career by the following methods (as outlined by Abbott, Pelc, & Mercier, 2019): (1) self-reflecting on one's own power, privilege, and marginalized identity status, including how this may change as we become more clinically experienced (as directed in the previous chapter, Guideline 1); (2) continuing to engage in learning about cultural nuances and practices throughout one's lifetime (as we explore more in Chapter/Guideline 4); (3) allowing trainees to evaluate which of their own and their clients' intersectional identity factors are most salient in the context of therapy; (4) creating a learning environment where cultural humility (and discussion about one's own missteps) can safely occur (as outlined in Chapter 9 on issues to consider within the context of supervision); (5) respecting and acknowledging your own trainees' cultural identities as they navigate therapy and supervision, and how these intersect with your own cultural biases and beliefs as a supervisor (again, covered in more detail in Chapter 9).

Research has supported the utility of such cultural humility practices in terms of establishing stronger therapeutic alliance (or even repairing ruptures) with clients (e.g., Owen et al., 2016). Case studies have highlighted how the integration of cultural humility principles into therapeutic settings can also improve engagement in therapy by clients from diverse backgrounds and facilitate retention in treatment (e.g., with first-generation college students; Rovitto, 2020). In this guideline we therefore explore the practical ways to take a culturally humble approach in our clinical practice, regardless of the specific treatment approach or problem area being targeted. Culturally humble supervisory practices and implementation are covered in Chapter 9, as that chapter specifically focuses on integrating our guidelines into the supervisory relationship with trainees.

In the rest of this chapter, let's first review what a cultural misstep might look like in the context of therapy using one of our case studies (Massie), and then review an exercise that guides you through a self-reflection on how to draw on your own cultural humility when such missteps occur, followed by an exercise on how to practice cultural humility and build awareness of potential microaggressions and missteps taken in therapy. I will then return to the case example provided and ask you to reflect on how you might repair any ruptures caused and model active practice of the cultural humility skill, before describing how this might look in practice with this particular client. The chapter will end with a reminder of how we can engage in that crucial life-long learning that is central to cultural humility as a core principle of good culturally competent therapy and a consideration of what might get in the way of that effort.

## CASE APPLICATION (PART 1)

*Case description.* Massie is a 46-year-old second-generation Filipinx-American, nonbinary individual who identifies as bisexual, and who is recently divorced after coming out to their family. They are currently a single parent of two teenage children, and they identify strongly with their Catholic faith, which causes significant distress and conflict with their sexual orientation (which they have otherwise come to terms with). They present with symptoms that appear to be consistent with major depression and generalized anxiety disorder, with their primary reported complaints being anhedonia, difficulty with staying asleep, overeating, often worrying about daily events, their family relationships, and their future romantic relationships, which comes with significant muscle tension/backaches, concentration difficulties, and significant irritability with their children. They also endorse occasional passive suicidal ideation ("what's the point of being here?"), but stated they would never consider killing themselves because of a fear of the after-life consequences for doing so, based on their faith. From the initial assessment, it seems that their family and faith/cultural communities are mixed in their reactions to their recently disclosed sexual orientation; their children have no issue with it, although the children are upset over the divorce. Their parents seem supportive, but their extended family members and certain members of their church are very vocal about both their divorce and various queer identities as being perceived as sinful.

*Preamble to therapy dialogue.* The therapist treating Massie was a 42-year-old cis-gendered female therapist who had immigrated from South Asia as a young adult, and who had been in an academic specialty clinic for about 15 years since receiving her clinical degree. The therapist was assigned to Massie as their clinician based on the therapist's expertise in treating their primary symptoms, and her own identification as an Asian minority and similar age to the client. Knowing the potential cultural match based on their similar age and similar Asian cultural heritages where family connections and collectivist approaches are highly valued, the therapist had established a decent alliance with Massie in the first few sessions. However, in session 4, as the client was starting to engage in more intensive cognitive restructuring and behavioral activation (the evidence-based approach taken with this case, as we discuss in more detail in Chapter/Guideline 7 when we also revisit this case), the therapist commits a cultural misstep and microaggression by misgendering the client in front of a colleague, as described in the following excerpt from their work together.

**Therapist** [greeting client in waiting room to lead them back to her office]: *Hi Massie, good to see you! Ready to begin? Come on back with me.*

As they start to go down the hallway away from the waiting room toward the therapist's office, they are briefly stopped by another clinician in the hallway wishing to talk to the therapist, who doesn't at first realize that the therapist is walking with a client.

**Therapist**: *Oh, sorry, I can't chat about that administrative issue right now [motioning to Massie], my client and I are about to start our session. When she and I are all done with our session, I'll come find you, okay?*

Massie noticeably bristles at hearing the misgendered pronoun the therapist uses, and their smile from greeting the therapist disappears. The therapist does not notice or immediately realize her misstep, but does note that as soon as they enter her office moments later and the client sits across from her, that they look visibly upset and show guarded body language.

Following this clear and detectable shift in affect during the session, the therapist was keenly aware that something had ruptured in the therapeutic alliance with the client, but was struggling with detecting what exactly happened because she misgendered the client so automatically that it was not immediately apparent to her. She found herself caught between feeling like she should move forward with the agreed-upon and protocol-determined agenda for the session, and a desire to address the rupture, but not knowing how to do so while not being clear on what that misstep was. She opted to start with setting the agenda and going into homework review as her typical first step, and as the client stiffly and reluctantly started to share their progress with their homework goals, the therapist suddenly realized that she used "she" instead of the client's correct (and previously clearly stated preference) for the pronoun "they" in the hallway. The therapist feels both mortified and embarrassed at this mistake, and conflicted about whether now to interrupt the homework review since the client has not raised the issue themselves. The therapist is now also second-guessing herself whether this is the misstep that has occurred, even though she detects continuing reticence from Massie.

Such a multilayered and complex set of reactions or competing demands in the face of a therapeutic rupture is not unusual. If you have encountered any type of rupture in therapeutic alliance (whether due to a cultural misstep or not), you have firsthand experience about how challenging this can be to navigate. Thus, self-reflection here is key, and to be clear, it is okay (particularly in the beginning practice of cultural humility) for such self-reflection to occur after the session, with some distance and space from the rupture. Over time, it will become easier to compress the steps for such self-reflection, as outlined in Exercise 2.1 ("Self-Reflection after a Therapeutic Rupture or Cultural Misstep Occurs"), and it will start to happen more in "real time" as we gain more practice and self-awareness over years of experience.

Exercise 2.1

## SELF-REFLECTION AFTER A THERAPEUTIC RUPTURE OR CULTURAL MISSTEP OCCURS

Consider the following questions to explore the therapeutic rupture, and use the spaces provided to **write your answers** for each to fully reflect on the situation.

1. Even before getting into the specifics of content of the misstep, explore: How do I know I made a possible cultural misstep or committed a microaggression? How did affect in the room change, and what did that feel like? Was the client noticeably distressed/angry/sad/withdrawn, or was it subtler? Was it more about how I felt that cued me in to what happened?

   a. Ways I noticed that I made a misstep or performed a microaggression:

   *************************************************************

2. What were the sequences of events/interactions leading up to the noticeable shift in affect or visible emotional reaction from my client? That is, what was the exact nature/content of my misstep?

   a. Sequence of events leading to rupture:

   b. Content or nature of the cultural misstep:

   *************************************************************

3. What happened right after the rupture seems to have occurred, in terms of changes to the therapeutic alliance and session content? What is the likely impact of this rupture on future sessions and longer-term alliance with the client?

   a. Immediate consequences of the misstep/rupture:

   b. Possible long-term consequences of the misstep/rupture on therapeutic alliance/ability to meet therapeutic goals:

   *************************************************************

4. What are possible interpretations or internal reactions experienced by the client due to my misstep, based on (1) my understanding of their overall life experiences (e.g., other discriminatory experiences they have shared in session); (2) due to specific identity-related factors that they have expressed as salient/important to them; and (3) based on our own power-privilege differential in the therapist-client relationship?

   a. Possible interpretations/reactions by client:

   b. Client life experiences that may have contributed to their negative reaction to my misstep:

   c. Salient/important identity factors for client that were threatened by my misstep:

   d. Specific power or privilege differentials between my client and me that could enhance a negative reaction to my misstep:

   **************************************************************

5. What did I feel internally as I committed the misstep, in terms of physical feelings and emotions? What thoughts were going through my head then? And how did I behaviorally react/what did I do if the misstep was immediately noticeable to me?

   a. Physical feelings when I realized I committed the misstep or I noticed a shift in alliance:

   b. Emotions:

   c. Thoughts:

   d. Behaviors:

After this vulnerable and authentic self-reflection around what occurred leading up to the observed rupture, the therapist would be able to further come to terms with what parts of this rupture were directly due to the therapist's own cultural gaps in knowledge. Specifically, such a reflection would hopefully lead to an acknowledgment by the therapist that while she regarded herself as culturally competent, that she was less versed in working with clients identifying as gender diverse, and struggled even in her personal life with consistently sticking to a wider diversity of preferred pronouns due to little exposure stemming from her own cultural background. The therapist also could use this exercise to explore whether she was biased toward nonbinary individuals because of her own unfamiliarity and challenges with different pronoun use, and to focus on doing her own diversity training work to address such biases. Through this reflection, the therapist would be better positioned to more effectively shift her focus to addressing the misstep and repairing the therapeutic rupture.

To repair the misstep in a culturally humble way, Exercise 2.2 ("Repairing Cultural Missteps and Actively Practicing Cultural Humility") outlines a schema for actively addressing the strain on the therapeutic relationship caused by a therapist's cultural misstep or microaggression in order to rebuild alliance and partnership as an important precursor to continuing with the evidence-based treatment. This effort is important to minimize impacts of the misstep on the effectiveness of the chosen EBP and to maximize the client's benefit from therapy. First, it can be very useful to engage one's peers and supervisors in a frank conversation about what occurred, how your client reacted, how you felt, and what impact it already had or may have in the future on your work together. Doing so helps the therapist process what exactly occurred and potentially reduces the likelihood of such a misstep from reoccurring given the focus on all parts of the incident.

Exercise 2.2

## Repairing Cultural Missteps and Actively Practicing Cultural Humility

These are some ways to garner your sense of cultural humility and address cultural missteps or microaggressions you have committed toward others, which should be explored after thorough self-reflection, as outlined in Exercise 2.1.

1. **Engage** your peers and supervisors in an open, honest discussion about your reflections about the misstep that occurred, in terms of what occurred, the client's reactions, your reactions, probable impacts on the therapeutic alliance, and possible threats to the therapeutic agenda. This includes sharing vulnerable feelings of internalized biases, your own societal messaging or life experiences underlying your committed misstep to better articulate and explicitly name your own cultural gaps in knowledge. A tip for supervisors/peers receiving this reflection: Share your own examples of missteps or relevant experiences that put you at risk for committing a microaggression, including your own power/privilege status with a trainee, to model this openness and crucial vulnerability in the cultural humility process.

2. **Strategize** with supervisors and peers about how you can raise the misstep directly and explicitly with the client in your next session, based on the client's own cultural background, interaction style, and specific symptoms that may intersect with such direct discussion. Explore how owning up to this mistake or explicitly addressing such a misstep with your client makes you feel, and how this fits into your own overall development as a therapist.

3. **Try** role-playing how you will raise and address the cultural misstep/microaggression with supervisors or colleagues prior to your session for practice. Think of adapting one of these statements:

   * *X, before we get started with our session agenda for today, I just wanted to raise something that happened last week that has been on my mind. Specifically, I want to apologize for when I said/did XYZ last week, and I am sorry if that was hurtful to you.*
   * As your therapist, I always strive to provide the most open, accepting, and safe environment for you to reach your goals, and by doing XYZ [be explicit, no excuses!], I violated that promise of such a safe space. That is not in line with my professional values, and I am truly sorry that I behaved in such a way. I felt [shame, guilt, anger at myself, sadness] by how I behaved/ what I said.

* *Would you be open to sharing how you felt or what you thought when I said/ did XYZ? What was that like for you?*
* *How can I rebuild your trust or help you feel comfortable and accepted/ safe in session moving forward? I think we have already had a lot of positive progress toward your goals of ABC, and I want to do whatever I can to make sure my mistake does not move us away from continuing to achieve your goals.* [Be ready with a few ways you can suggest on your own, if your client isn't sure, so it doesn't fall all on them].

4. **Be brave and address your misstep** with your client by doing what you practiced with others. This is your final step of learning cultural humility, and trust me—it gets easier and becomes more second-nature with repeated practice!

Following this, the therapist can actively strategize possible ways to address the misstep with the client with the assistance of peers or supervisors, based on both the client's and the therapist's own cultural backgrounds, interaction styles, and the client's specific symptoms that may intersect with elements of power and privilege with such direct or explicit discussion of the misstep. For instance, certain cultures (e.g., individualistic cultures) might value a more direct approach to recounting the event and might not negatively judge such admission of fault by the therapist, or the client (regardless of their cultural background) might appreciate such a direct addressing of a microaggression because of what they have shared about their previous experiences of discrimination. Alternatively, if a client has specific clinical symptoms such as social anxiety, they may be more reticent to engage in any direct confrontation, and therefore the approach might have to be gentler and softer in the way the topic is raised, although this is not a reason to not own up or address one's missteps. Even a client who does not prefer direct confrontation or is uncomfortable with others' discomfort could benefit from such a modeling of how one can be vulnerable and how to take responsibility for actions that hurt others. Therefore, this is likely not only to address the rupture, but also could be beneficial therapeutically for the client.

Next, therapists of all experience levels are encouraged to role-play the agreed-upon approach; Exercise 2.2 provides some sample prompts. Practicing beforehand (with others, or in a mirror if you don't have colleagues/supervisors readily available) can increase your comfort with raising such a difficult incident and allow you to navigate your own relationship to the power differential with your client to bring your most authentic, culturally humble presence to the interaction. The last step is to actually do it—own up, practice tolerating the difficult emotions that are likely to come up when you do, and know that, like all the skills we learn as therapists, it will become easier with practice.

## CASE APPLICATION (PART 2)

So now let's return to our therapist and Massie, to see how the therapist exemplified this skill of repairing a misstep in the following dialogue. Here, as the therapist is more skilled with addressing cultural missteps more broadly, and because of her own prior self-reflection around her lack of familiarity with gender-diverse individuals, she addresses the misstep right at the beginning of the session, using step 4 from Exercise 2.2 (followed by steps 1–3 after the session, as described after the exchange below), choosing to pause the homework review to do so.

**Therapist**: *Massie, thank you for starting to describe some of the homework we assigned in session last week around noticing your negative automatic thoughts and starting to categorize some of the potential thinking traps in each. If we could actually pause on that for a moment, I want to just turn our attention to something more pressing. I noticed as soon as we came in here that you seem to be uncomfortable or upset. I also noticed as I sat down and we started* *homework review that I made a terrible mistake in the hallway when we were coming in here, and I want to know if those two things are connected. I just realized that I misgendered you and referred to you as "she" with my colleague instead of "they." I am so sorry for this—it was not my intention to use the incorrect pronoun when I know how much your gender identity has been a source of stress for you and how important this part of your identity is for you. Regardless of my intention, I can only imagine this was upsetting for you. Am I totally off base in guessing that you are feeling upset and this is the reason why? If there is another reason altogether, I want to hear about that, too, if you're willing to share.*

**Massie:** *No, you're right. That was really difficult to hear, but it's fine, I don't want to talk about it. I'm used to being called the wrong pronoun, it's just disappointing for it to happen here.*

**Therapist:** *I don't think it's fine—I am also very disappointed in myself for making such a mistake, and making you feel at all that this is not a safe place where every part of your identity is respected and celebrated. I have some work to do on myself and in my work with you to make sure I can make up for this. I want to continue to show you that this is a space where you can receive the type of treatment that shows that the way you identify, on all fronts, is valued and matters. I definitely don't want to push you to talk about it if you don't want to, but I also want you to know that this is a space where we can talk about it, where you can tell me if I ever make you feel devalued or mislabeled, and we can work together to address that. I also promise to continue to be transparent in our work together to share how I'm making efforts to ensure I don't make such a mistake in our work together again. Is there anything I can do right now to make up for my mistake?*

**Massie:** *I don't think so. I do appreciate you brought it up, that makes me feel a bit better already, although I'm still a bit ruffled. I think the best thing for me is if you promise to continue working on that, not just for me, but for so many queer people who are constantly misgendered, and a therapist particularly shouldn't be one who makes someone feel upset in that way. Otherwise, I'd just like to continue to get help on my depression, which is what I came here for.*

**Therapist:** *I totally respect that. I agree that this is an area I need to work on so I make sure I don't make this mistake again, and I will be doing some self-reflection and additional training to work on this part of my service, both out of my respect for you and, as you so nobly said, for the queer community in general. Again, I completely agree that therapy should be a safe place free from such mistreatment, and you are absolutely justified in feeling upset with me as a result. Thank you for being so kind as to engage me in this discussion to make me a better person and therapist, and I promise to at least make this experience one that strengthens our therapy relationship together. Let's return to your homework review, and work on our planned skills to tackle your depression today.*

*Summary of guideline application.* Thus, as exemplified by this exchange, the therapist immediately and directly owns her misstep and explicitly names it (e.g., saying "I misgendered you" versus something vague like "I said something that wasn't quite right or was hurtful to you"). It is important to be clear about what your misstep specifically was, to show acknowledgment for how hurtful it could be and why. The therapist also, even with some minimization from the client, still shares her own reaction to the misstep, not invalidating the client's experience (note how she says, "I don't think it's fine," versus "No, you should be more upset, it's objectively not fine"), thus modeling even here that each of them can have feelings that are strong and differ, and the therapist can do wrong, which directly targets the power differential in the room to create a space where the client feels like they can then subsequently say, "Okay, you're right, that was not okay" if they feel that to be the case. The therapist makes a promise to address her own deficiencies in this regard and to be open about her process as relevant to the client, and then respects the client's wishes to just return to treatment.

Now, either in this session or a future one, the therapist might decide to actually use this misgendering incident as part of their current cognitive restructuring work, asking the client if they noticed any automatic thoughts when the incident occurred, and potentially helping the client see how such events continue to contribute to their own depression outside of therapy, but this should be done with discretion, when the client looks ready to accept that (given they seem reticent in this exchange to talk much about it) and the rupture has been a bit more repaired. After the session, the therapist proceeded to engage her peers at her clinical center and even used what happened as a teaching tool with her supervisees to model cultural humility when one makes such missteps and to generate solutions with the team about what she could have done in addition and ways to avoid such missteps in the future, following the remaining steps 1–3 in Exercise 2.2.

This process of actively practicing cultural humility could be followed for any number of potential cultural missteps that commonly occur within the context of therapy, the major categories of which are outlined in Table 2.1. Specifically, common cultural missteps tend to fall into some major categories. First, one major category includes the performance of microaggressions (as exemplified by the misgendering example in the case study), which can involve either verbal slights/insults based on specific identity facets toward a client, nonverbal behaviors that reflect discriminatory actions based on a client's background, or use of stereotypical terms when referring to clients with others. Another major category of cultural missteps occurs in case conceptualization, whereby the therapist starts to conflate their own value system with what the client should be striving for, whether that's setting life goals that align with one's own family or relationship values as the therapist, or personal beliefs about agency or the value of individualism/collectivism, or categorizing a client as fully a product of their identity background, or ignoring these facets altogether.

Finally, the way we interact with clients, even if insult or stereotyping is unintentional, can be the culprit of another category of cultural missteps. For instance, ways we talk with clients about their own communication styles (e.g., pointing

*Table 2.1* COMMON CULTURAL MISSTEPS

| Microaggressions | Case Conceptualization | Interaction Style |
|---|---|---|
| Maltreatment of clients directly based on their identity (race/ethnicity, culture, gender, sexual orientation, disability status etc.) | Conflating one's own value systems/beliefs/ biases with clinical conceptualization of maintaining symptoms and subsequent goals for treatment | Unintentionally interacting in ways with clients that emphasize their difference in identity from you or the "mainstream" culture, effectively "othering" the client over repeated interactions |
| • Verbal insults (e.g., using offensive or incorrect terms, mispronunciation of names)<br>• Nonverbal discriminatory behaviors (e.g., guarded body language, disapproving facial expressions)<br>• Use of stereotypical tropes when describing clients in context of clinical supervision or clinical reports (e.g., "as is typical for African people . . .") | • Superimposing our own values about ideal family systems and interpersonal dynamics in therapy targets for clients (e.g., how close children should be to their parents or should move out of their family home, what romantic relationships should look like)<br>• Incorporating our own beliefs in treatment targets when not raised by client (e.g., pushing clients to espouse feminist values, encouraging clients to solely align with individualistic values)<br>• Assuming that a client completely adheres to their cultural or identity background practices or only to their individually-valued practices, instead of a combination of both | • Comments about the client's own communication (e.g., repeatedly noting difficulties in understanding their accent, or asking about where they are from if they don't readily share)<br>• Use of categorizing terms that actively separate them from us as the therapists (e.g., "your community," "where you come from," instead of directly naming their community such as "being Arab American")<br>• Specifically avoiding engaging in any appropriate levels of self-disclosure about your own identity/background, thereby solidifying a power/privilege boundary, particularly where these concepts are already quite salient |

out accents or pushing for details on cultural background) and the ways we refer to their individual experiences (e.g., using terms such as "your community," or "your background") instead of actually using the terms that are more precise in what we're referring to, such as their specific community name or utilized cultural terms can result in an "othering" process with our clients, which can unravel therapeutic alliance over time. Similarly, while self-disclosure is not an explicit prescription in really any of the EBPs we use, adopting this into your interaction style with clients can model cultural humility and openness to the bidirectionality of the therapy process. Conversely, avoiding such disclosure about your own background or obvious differences in identity facets between you and a client can result in an inauthentic interaction style and can solidify perceived power and privilege differentials that exist within the client-therapist dyad.

## COMMON CHALLENGES

Again, while I'm fairly sure we agree that the ability to be culturally humble and open to admitting one's missteps is a crucial part of being just a competent therapist more broadly, this skill is not an easy one to develop or practice. To start, it takes considerable self-attunement and situational awareness to notice the nuanced verbal and subtle nonverbal cues that others provide when we inadvertently make a cultural misstep in the context of therapy or supervision, and ruptures in alliance stemming from such missteps may be hard to detect if we miss some of these reactionary signs from others (see Box 2.1).

Further, when we do detect our own cultural missteps, it is common to either feel defensive about the impact or importance of that misstep for the therapeutic alliance, or to feel shame/embarrassment at having caused such a rupture in the first place. Either emotional reaction can have similar consequences; we are less likely to address the misstep and engage avoidance of raising it in the context of therapy or supervision, either because of our own minimization of the impact of the misstep or out of our own discomfort in revealing our vulnerability as

---

Box 2.1

### Common Challenges in Implementing Guideline 2

* Missing verbal and (subtle) nonverbal cues from clients about when a cultural misstep or rupture has occurred in therapy due to over-attention to treatment protocol at hand
* Feelings of shame or embarrassment at having committed a misstep leading to avoidance of correcting or addressing its consequences
* Feeling defensive about the impact or significance of a cultural misstep from clients, supervisors, or even in reaction to one's own emotional reaction to this realization
* Uncertainty about how to adequately and inoffensively address the misstep that leaves you feeling unable to address it altogether

---

therapists (who typically hold a place of expertise in the therapy relationship and who create the space for vulnerability in a unidirectional way from client to therapist, not the other way around).

As a last major challenge to our practice of cultural humility in the therapy or supervision context, even if we wish to address the issue, we often don't know how to effectively do so, in a way that does not cause further harm. Indeed, this is often reported as a major challenge to being culturally humble in my cultural competency trainings. This is not a minor issue, because it is one thing to be taught to address cultural missteps with a listing of concrete steps to help you do so, and it's another to experientially feel all the emotions that come with verbalizing a mistake, absorbing the shift in affect in the therapy room from making such a misstep explicit, and accepting the consequences that come with such a process of committing, owning up to, and attempting to smooth over such missteps with clients.

In these ways, practicing cultural humility is really hard; making a misstep that hurts or offends our clients is the precise *opposite* of what we strive for in a therapeutic context. Thus, when such a misstep occurs, and we are aware of it, we must work through a number of additional layers that extend beyond other types of ruptures related to noncompliance or resistance to our core therapeutic strategies, including our own resistance, strong emotions such as shame, and really, a violation to our likely long-standing beliefs about our own infallibility as therapists or as nonbiased, fair individuals more generally. In the next section, I provide some guidance around ways we might practice cultural humility, summarizing ways for us to address a misstep, as exemplified both in the case study, Exercise 2.2, and from other points discussed in this chapter.

## PUTTING IT INTO PRACTICE

As delineated in Box 2.2., our practice of this particular skill of cultural humility has two branches, depending on the situation. In the first, we are either clearly aware that we did, said, or behaved in an offensive or biased way toward a client, or at least have strong suspicions that we did. If this is the case, there are some clear steps we can follow, as outlined by experts in the field and from my own clinical experience around when cultural missteps occur within the context of therapy. First, self-reflection continues to be a key factor. Supervisors, peers, and even our support systems outside of our professional roles may be able to observe or describe ways in which our own biases may cloud our behavior in therapy, but that ability to sit with ourselves and to practice vulnerability around our weaknesses, shortcomings, and cultural blind spots as clinicians is crucial. Exercise 2.1, reviewed earlier in the context of the case study, can be a useful way to engage ourselves in such self-reflection, and importantly, repeated self-reflection in this way will increase our own tolerance to feeling vulnerable as therapists and improve our ability to detect shifts in therapeutic alliance or our own cultural missteps in therapy over time.

Box 2.2

## How Do I Practice Guideline 2?

When you are aware that a misstep likely occurred:

1. **Reflect** on how the session went to work through the chain of events that led to the rupture (hint: look at Exercise 2.1).
2. **Practice authenticity and vulnerability** with yourself to notice how the interaction felt to you and what it likely caused for the client.
3. **Consult** about the misstep with supervisors/peers to receive support and a sounding board for how it should be addressed/raised with client.
4. **Explicitly raise** the misstep in the next session with client (see Exercise 2.2); be ready to **revisit** this misstep and how it impacts future interactions.
5. **Continue practicing** being attuned to your client's reactions and your own language, biases, and reactions to their diversity markers in session to reduce likelihood of such missteps.

When you are unclear whether a misstep occurred or have a hard time detecting it:

6. **Enlist the help** of a clinical supervisor or clinical peer/fellow therapist to review the chain of events (either through actual recorded snippets of session or a recounting of content) to obtain external feedback on antecedents and consequences of the interaction and whether a misstep might have occurred.
7. If it is likely that a misstep occurred with such review and consultation, **work through steps 1–5 in Exercise 2.1.**

---

Following such a self-reflection and exposure to the emotions stemming from this reflection (whether that is shame, guilt, anger, and even defensiveness), it is important to get peer and/or supervisory support. As a reminder, I provide some guidance in Chapter 9 on what the supervisor is advised to do to build a training atmosphere that is nonjudgmental and open to such reflections by modeling accountability of one's own mistakes. Assuming this exists, the next step is to seek consultation with one's supervisor or peers about what occurred from your perspective and to discuss what likely went on for the client and how this may impact alliance and efforts toward therapeutic recovery or the EBP being utilized. This should lead to an exploration around how to address the misstep in therapy with the client, with a consideration for how to balance making space for this important deviation from the treatment, while not threatening the intervention agenda or core components.

After such careful self-reflection and consultation, it is now important to raise the misstep with the client directly. As outlined in Exercise 2.2 and the Case Application, this effort includes several key elements, including owning up (and being explicit) about the misstep that occurred, taking full responsibility for it (no excuses), exploring how the client felt about it, and gauging the extent to which they would like to discuss it, committing to improving this area of competency, and continuing to check in about the impact of the misstep on the alliance or as a means to work on therapeutic skills at a future session when the client is ready to receive that. Importantly, remember that a rupture due to a cultural misstep, similar to other sources of therapeutic ruptures, are not accomplished with one attempt to address. You must be ready to revisit the impact of this on future interactions with clients, and we must remember to continue being attuned to our interactions with the client (including continued self-reflection on our language use, reactions, and internalized biases to their identity markers) to minimize repeated offenses in the cultural context.

An alternative branch to the practice of cultural humility is when we do not even detect that a cultural misstep or therapeutic rupture has occurred. My hope is that some of the exercises and examples in this chapter will help you increase your own self-awareness and attunement to others so that this pathway is less traveled over time as we all develop as therapists. However, if this is the case for you, it is helpful to periodically share how therapy is progressing with different clients with either a supervisor or peer. With a supervisor, while review of clients' progress and therapy session content is already being conducted, it is useful to make the interactions around cultural nuances and wording the focus of review periodically, to obtain external feedback on how we are performing from a cultural competency and equitable treatment perspective. The review can be of actual recorded portions of a session (if allowable by a client), or by one's recounting of distinct interactions with a client where maybe even we detected a shift in alliance or "pulling away" of the client, even if we can't detect a cultural misstep as being the source of such a shift. And if with consultation it is determined that a cultural misstep likely occurred, we can work ourselves through the steps in the first branch of practicing cultural humility as described previously.

While none of these steps can give you complete certainty that a cultural misstep will be repaired and treatment effectiveness will not be irrevocably threatened, our efforts in this regard to actively, consciously, and genuinely improve our cultural humility will assist us in continuing to be the best therapists we can be. And, it does get easier to go through these steps over time, as daunting as it can seem at first!

## COMMENTARY ON INCORPORATING SOCIAL JUSTICE

As someone who has personally and professionally experienced multiple instances of invalidation based on one or more of my identity factors (whether due to my gender, race, or immigrant status), I have also been in the role not only of the oppressed, but certainly also of the oppressor (even if unintentionally so). My own specific intersection of power and privilege have continually (and dynamically) interacted with my own facets of identity; thus, cultural humility and awareness of my responsibility to ensure that others are treated equitably have been long intertwined and fairly inescapable for me. I do not claim that these two concepts go in hand in hand for everyone; each individual has their own valid and unique lived experience. Rather, I implore you to think about how the cultivation and practice of cultural humility intersect with your own efforts to create a socially just mental health space for those we serve and our communities at large. I predict that for most of us, some reflection on these two concepts and how they reasonably play out in each of our current clinical practices will lead us to similar conclusions that being culturally humble is directly linked to a commitment to socially just practice. Thus, ensuring this skill is honed and continually prioritized in our careers serves a dual purpose to individual clients and to addressing health disparities more broadly.

## DISCUSSION QUESTIONS

1. What do you think about the suitability of the phrase "cultural humility" to capture the process of addressing cultural missteps and admitting to one's diversity-related gaps in knowledge? What other constructs or descriptions capture this skill better, if you are not in favor of this term?

2. What are some concrete ways in which we can practice cultural humility across our professional roles (e.g., in clinical situations, teaching/mentoring, research, administrative/leadership responsibilities)?

3. What are some examples of your own cultural missteps with others in one or more professional domains? How did you address these missteps, and how would you address them if they occurred again now?

4. Think of one way you could practice cultural humility professionally or personally *today*. What do you notice around your emotions and thoughts about taking such action? How can you manage those internal reactions and still commit to practicing this skill in the way you thought of?

5. **Social Justice Action**: How may we apply a cultural humility approach to broader public health policy and/or institutional processes (e.g., hiring, supervision, teaching) involving advocacy around improved inclusion, access, and equity issues?

# 3

# Guideline 3

## *Balancing Culturally Informed and Individualized Assessment of the Presenting Problem*

### GUIDELINE 3 EXPLAINED

While it is tempting to jump into using cultural modifications based on an assumption that a client's salient identity factors have a strong influence on their presenting problems, many in the field agree that this is not the recommended course of action (Asnaani & Hofmann, 2012). In fact, automatically adopting a modified treatment based solely on the fact that the client identifies from a particular identity facet is regarded as premature and potentially problematic (Sue & Zane, 2009). In short, some of the foundational skills of assessment (i.e., examining the exact nature of the presenting problem and all contributing factors, which may include cultural or diversity-related issues) are applicable to cases from *all* backgrounds, and completely in line with good culturally informed assessment practice. Regardless of one's stated alignment with particular identity-based groups, each client should still be acknowledged as a unique individual with their own variable level of impact of various identity factors on the psychological issues they are seeking treatment for, and it is important to understand that there is heterogeneity in dominance or influence of diversity-related factors even within a particular identity group.

Thus, a cornerstone element of engaging in culturally responsive treatment lies within adequate, culturally informed (but person-specific) assessment of the client's concerns. For instance, it is important to ask about cultural beliefs not only to establish trust and openness in the therapy setting, but also to explicitly assess how (and whether) those beliefs specifically shape, inform, or maintain the psychological symptoms for which the client is presenting to therapy. It is important not to automatically assume that a stated cultural belief or value (which just might be raised due to these being personally meaningful to a client) is connected to their reported emotional health symptoms, just as it is unadvisable to ignore or

*A Cultural Humility and Social Justice Approach to Psychotherapy.* Anu Asnaani, Oxford University Press.
© Oxford University Press 2023. DOI: 10.1093/oso/9780197635971.003.0004

omit questions related to cultural beliefs or values because they do not appear to be related to reported symptoms at face value.

So, how do we find the balance of not assuming too much, and yet not asking enough? Herein lies an important lesson that we have learned as more of us engage in work with individuals from a range of diverse and intersectional identity backgrounds: do good assessment, and do the same for everyone, regardless of their "visible" identities. For instance, one routine way to ensure that something is assessed adequately in the identity domain (particularly as it relates to the emotional target symptoms) is to incorporate two to four questions on this topic within your typical assessment battery, whether that entails a standardized semi-structured diagnostic interview or an unstructured assessment procedure. These additions should be standard practice and included for *all* clients, not just those identifying with a minoritized identity. As shown in Box 3.1, there are a few simple questions that could be incorporated at various points of the assessment sessions, which allow you to ascertain (1) the identity factors most valued by or salient to a client; (2) the client's perspective on how relevant these stated identity factors are to their current symptoms for which they are seeking treatment; and (3) the client's willingness to address or incorporate their cultural beliefs and values into the presented evidence-based practice (EBP) or treatment plan.

---

Box 3.1

SAMPLE PROMPTS TO ASSESS FOR THE IMPACT OF IDENTITY FACTORS ON THE PRESENTING PROBLEM

This is by no means an exhaustive list, but it will hopefully get you started on thinking about how to raise identity-related influences within your assessment of the presenting problem. These prompts can also be posed to clients for continuous case conceptualization at various points over the course of therapy, not just at the beginning of treatment.

Note: If you're using a semi-structured standardized assessment/diagnostic interview, you can also add the following questions to round out your assessment and ensure you are examining the influence of identity factors within this more structured context. Depending on your practice policies, you just may not be able to ask as many follow-up questions and may be required to leave this for the first therapy sessions. Regardless, it's important to at least mention the first stem to open up the space for the client to discuss these issues.

* [FOLLOWING PSYCHOSOCIAL HISTORY AND EVALUATION OF CHIEF COMPLAINT]: *Thank you for providing information on why you are seeking services and telling me a little bit about your life outside of your most troubling symptoms. One last thing I wanted to raise was that you mentioned that* [XYZ identity factor] *is important to you* [OR] *that you identify as* [XYZ identity factor], *and I just wanted to understand whether you think that being*

[XYZ identity factor] *influences the main symptoms of* [specific disorder] *we talked about today? This could be both in terms of how these identities make your symptoms worse, but also if you think they help you cope with your symptoms better.*

* [FOLLOW-UP TO THIS PREVIOUS QUESTION IF CLIENT IS UNSURE WHAT YOU MEAN]: *So, what I mean is that often individuals coming into our clinic will mention that they identify with a particular race, religion, gender, or even specific community. Since we are more than our mental health symptoms, we like to know about how our clients identify in these other ways so we can understand you as a person more fully. Also, sometimes those very identities (or a combination of them) can impact the mental health symptoms we are trying to help you target in therapy, either in positive ways (like giving you a healthy way to cope with feeling depressed or lonely, for example) or in negative ways (like feeling down about how your symptoms affect your community or are not in line with your community's values), or even a combination. Do you think your identity influences anything we have spoken about so far today? It is totally fine if it does not, but I just want to make sure I do not miss something important that might be part of what is going on for you or that may help us come up with the most useful treatment plan.*

* [IF CLIENT ENDORSES INFLUENCE OF IDENTITY FACTOR(S) ON CURRENT TREATMENT-SEEKING, ASK THEM TO TELL YOU AS MUCH AS THEY ARE COMFORTABLE DOING, AND THEN]: *Thank you so much for sharing that insight on how being* [XYZ identity factor, explicitly stated, avoid using generalities] *might have an influence on the symptoms that brought you into the assessment today. We will likely come back to this discussion throughout the therapy periodically to continue to explore how these identity factors continue to play a role. But you can also feel free to bring these up any time over the course of your treatment with us, this is always a welcome space to do so.*

* [IF CLIENT DENIES ANY INFLUENCE/RELEVANCE OF IDENTITY FACTORS]: *That's completely fine if you do not think how you identify* [or being XYZ] *has a significant impact on what we have discussed so far in terms of your mental health symptoms. If that changes, and you want to raise the discussion again in the future over the course of your treatment with us, I just want you to know that there is always a welcome space to do so here.*

* [FOLLOW-UP CHECK-IN AT FUTURE SESSIONS ABOUT INFLUENCE OF IDENTITY FACTORS]: *If you might recall, when we first were trying to figure out your main symptoms and what we wanted to target in the beginning of treatment, we discussed how being* [XYZ identity factor] *might be related to what we're targeting in treatment, in either helpful or unhelpful ways. I remember that at that time, we discussed that your symptoms were impacted in terms of* [FILL IN FROM PREVIOUS DISCUSSIONS] [OR] *did not feel impacted by these identities at the time. I'm curious whether this feels any different right now, and if so, how? What do you think the impact of being* [XYZ identity factor] *is on your symptoms at the current time?*

If time is an issue or you feel that you need some supplementation to what you can gather from the client directly as you are just starting to establish the alliance, then you certainly can also consider including any number of self-report measures in your symptom battery (if you use one for baseline and outcome measurement) that assess for one's cultural values and associated beliefs about seeking mental health treatment, importance of connection to others, discrimination experiences, and acculturation or immigration status, among others. See Table 3.1 for some examples of validated measures for this purpose, many of which are brief, available in multiple languages, and already tested with various racial/ethnic, cultural, and sexual minority groups, but which you can certainly consider applying to other identity factors (e.g., gender minorities, lower SES, being from a rural setting) where appropriate and indicated, to get a sense of the client's perspective on such issues.

*Table 3.1* SAMPLE STANDARDIZED ASSESSMENT MEASURES

| Self-Report Measures | Semi-Structured Interviews |
|---|---|
| **Discrimination measures:**<br>Everyday Discrimination Scale (EDS)<br>(Williams et al., 1997)<br>Detroit Area Study Discrimination Questionnaire<br>(Jackson & Williams, 2002) | **UConn Racial/Ethnic Stress and Trauma Survey (UnRESTS)**<br>(Williams, Metzger, Leins, & DeLapp, 2018)<br><br>* Specifically incorporates assessment of discrimination and racial trauma, using the CFI (see next) as the foundation |
| **Acculturative Stress:**<br>Multidimensional Acculturative Stress Inventory (MASI)<br>(Rodriguez, Myers, Mira, Flores, & Garcia-Hernandez, 2002)<br>Vancouver Acculturation Index (VIA)<br>(Ryder, Alden, & Paulhus, 2000) | ----------<br>**DSM-5 Cultural Formulation Interview (CFI)**<br>(American Psychiatric Association, 2013) |
| **Cultural Values/Orientation:**<br>Singelis Self-Construal scale (SCS)<br>(Singelis, 1994)<br>Culture Orientation Scale<br>(Triandis & Gelfland, 1998) | * Provides a cultural formulation integrated with DSM-5 diagnosis, found in appendix of DSM-5 |
| **Ethnic Identity:**<br>Multigroup Ethnic Identity Measure (MEIM)<br>(Roberts et al., 1999)<br>Ethnic Identity Scale (EIS)<br>(Umaña-Taylor, Yazedjian, & Bámaca-Gómez, 2004) | ----------<br>**Brief Cultural Interview (BCI)**<br>(Groen, Richters, Laban, & Devillé, 2017) |
| **Stigma toward mental health treatment:**<br>Self-Stigma of Seeking Help (SSOSH)<br>(Vogel, Wade, & Haake, 2006)<br>Stigma-9 Questionnaire (STIG-9)<br>(Gierk, Löwe, Murray, & Kohlmann, 2018) | * Primarily tested in immigrant/refugee populations in the Netherlands, at a more preliminary stage but shows promise given its brevity |

Finally, another core principle of good evidence-based assessment is that this process is a continuous one throughout the therapy relationship, and the concurrent evaluation of cultural or diversity-related factors and how they may impact treatment is certainly continuous as well. That is to say, while a client may not endorse a strong influence of identity factors early in treatment or at baseline assessment, this does not mean that these factors will not become more central to the work as treatment progresses. Thus, raising these issues and asking about them explicitly in the beginning allow the client to know that such questions can be explored and are not "off the table" for the work together, making it more comfortable for both the therapist and the client to raise identity-related factors throughout the course of treatment as the need arises.

In the rest of this chapter, let's examine how it might look to incorporate some of these important identity-based questions in a more unstructured assessment format within the context of the first few sessions with one of our case studies, Tess. As always, we'll conclude with some common challenges to such culturally informed yet individualized assessment, ways to practice this skill, and a review of the social justice components of this guideline.

## CASE APPLICATION

*Case description.* Tess is a 24-year-old Latina woman who immigrated from El Salvador as a teenager with her mother. She now lives near her uncle and his family in a major U.S. city, but she has several younger brothers and her father still living in El Salvador, all of whom she has not been able to see due to complications with her DACA immigration status. She presents to treatment with symptoms that seem most consistent with panic disorder with agoraphobia, specifically reporting sudden bouts of intense crying, acute anxiety, heat in the chest that radiates to her head, and significant avoidance of public places that she has deemed the most "risky" where such "emotion attacks" (as she calls them) are most likely to occur (e.g., supermarket, department stores, and when being on bridges). She has a good social circle consisting of both Latine and non-Latine friends, but often feels disconnected from her mother, who does not speak English and does not understand why Tess is pursuing a graduate degree in accounting, which causes significant tension in their relationship. Specifically, her mother is eager for Tess to enter the workforce to earn money so they may look at bringing the rest of their immediate family to the country, and Tess feels a lot of guilt around not helping her family in this way, but wants to make more money to support them in the future with a graduate degree.

*Evidence-based treatment approach.* Given Tess's chief complaints of panic symptoms and agoraphobia, the chosen treatment approach closely follows a front-line cognitive behavioral therapy (CBT) protocol for panic (such as that by Craske & Barlow, 2007). Specifically, this treatment includes provision of psychoeducation around the function of anxiety/panic, identifying unhelpful thoughts that may be maintaining the anxiety and subsequent avoidance (e.g., "these physical symptoms are harmful" or "being on bridges is unsafe because

I might panic"), and then coaching the client through the process of gradually approaching their feared situations via in vivo exposures, and building tolerance to unpleasant physical feelings of anxiety via interoceptive exposures (repeated, purposeful induction of physical symptoms of anxiety). Treatment typically occurs once a week for the standard session of 45–60 minutes for around 10–15 sessions.

*Preamble to therapy dialogue.* We examine the use of the strategies recommended by Guideline 3 within the context of the third session of therapy between Tess and her therapist. The initial intake showed that Tess reported perceived adaptive acculturation into the mainstream American culture, based on a psychosocial history that the client had a number of Spanish-speaking and non-Spanish-speaking friends, and was in graduate school, although there was familial guilt about not earning money and interpersonal conflict with her Spanish-speaking mother. The therapist is a 35-year-old, gay, Latino, cis-gendered man who was born and has been raised in the United States and is currently in a group private practice community setting.

As a seasoned community provider, this therapist is aware of how despite what might seem a shared cultural background, his experience of his Latine culture and the experience of Tess as a straight, cis-gendered woman and an immigrant are likely to be different, but he needs to assess the ways in which this might be the case. In their first two sessions, they have already covered some basic cultural history (e.g., understanding more about her immigration story and the emotions she feels around part of her family still being separated from her and her mother), along with significant psychoeducation around the function of anxiety and the reason why panic attacks may occur, in keeping with standard CBT for panic as described above. What he continues to be a bit unclear on is how much the stress related to her immigration status may be impacting her overall stress level and specific concerns when in supermarkets, stores, and on bridges (her main agoraphobic situations), and also how acculturated she is to these and other situational contexts based on her bicultural background. To shed some light on these issues, and to maximize his time in session with her, he has asked her to fill out the Multidimensional Acculturative Stress Inventory (MASI) (Rodriguez, Myers, Mira, Flores, & Garcia-Hernandez, 2002) and the Ethnic Identity Scale (EIS) (Umaña-Taylor, Yazedjian & Bámaca-Gómez, 2004) to obtain some insight into her levels of acculturation and ethnic identity-related stress (see Table 3.1), respectively. In the following dialogue with Tess in their third session together, the therapist utilizes some of the suggested prompts in this chapter and the findings from these self-report measures to better explore these cultural-level factors while trying to remain cognizant of how Tess's symptoms are individually being maintained for her.

**Therapist**: *Tess, before we get into fully understanding the rationale for exposure therapy today and creating what we call an exposure hierarchy to help you manage your panic symptoms, I wanted to chat with you a bit more about some of the parts of your story that are uniquely you, to see if they may be* *related to the work we're doing with your anxiety, and if so, how. I know we have already touched on this somewhat in previous sessions, but would that be okay to explore a bit more with you today?*

**Tess:** *I think so, yes. But what exactly do you want to talk about?*

**Therapist:** *Great, I'm glad you're open to it, and I'm very happy to elaborate. First, thank you for filling out those few extra measures today before session; those questionnaires were getting at some of the things I have been wondering about. Specifically, I'm sure you noticed that they asked a lot more about how stressful the immigrant experience and your current DACA status are for you, along with questions about how close you felt to Latino versus mainstream American culture. Does that sound like what the questions you answered were about?*

**Tess:** *Ah, yes. That is correct. But why would those things be important to discuss for my treatment of anxiety—do you think they are the reason I am panicking in the grocery store? I don't understand how those are related.*

**Therapist:** *I certainly don't know for sure if those types of things are connected to your panic symptoms. But I don't want us to miss out on exploring if they are, because they are a part of your history, and you have mentioned that your immigration story is a particularly big part of your life more generally. By chatting about it and giving ourselves space to explore the impact on being an immigrant or having to balance multiple cultures, we can figure out how much those two things are related to your feelings of panic and avoidance of certain situations. Does that make sense?*

**Tess:** *Okay. I don't think they are related because I immigrated a long time ago and these symptoms started only a few months ago, but I am open to talking a bit more about it to make sure.*

**Therapist:** *Perfect, and if it doesn't seem related, we can definitely put it to the side and only come back to it if it seems to be part of what we're working on here. I noticed in your questionnaire you mentioned feeling a fair level of negative emotions around being Latina and being from El Salvador. This seems quite consistent with what you have mentioned before. I'm just curious, has that stress around your Hispanic identity gone up at all recently?*

**Tess:** *No, it's always been that high, for at least a few years now since I became an adult.*

**Therapist:** *Okay, that's helpful to know, although I'm sorry that it's been so stressful for so long. That must be very difficult to have as a stressor for years on end, and I am here to support you with that any time you need to talk about it, whether or not it's related to our anxiety work. I'm curious, though, if I may ask a bit more about that one—have the other feelings you mentioned in session around feeling guilty about being in graduate school and not financially being able to help your mom and family back in El Salvador been more prevalent in the past few months or since starting graduate school?*

**Tess**: *Oh. I hadn't thought of that—I guess those thoughts have been much more frequent in the past 4–5 months or so, and the panic attacks did start shortly after beginning graduate school, yes. I just thought I was stressed from school, I didn't think it has to do with my guilt about my family.*

**Therapist**: *That's so insightful, Tess! That's really important that you noticed that the symptoms started soon after starting graduate school and you were chalking your higher anxiety up to the stress of school. And you know what, I think you are very much likely to be right about that—starting graduate school is stressful for many people, and it's not unusual to have an anxiety issue start soon after such a big life change. In your case, I'm wondering if the already stressful context of graduate school was further amplified because going to graduate school also meant disappointing your mom, who wanted you to work and start bringing in income, and also brought up additional guilt of not being able to financially support her and your family back home. Again, that might not fully be the case, but it might help us understand that your stress level was possibly high due to several factors, which as we discussed last week can trigger panic attacks more easily. What do you think of that possibility?*

**Tess**: *Hmm, I guess that's possible. I hadn't thought of it that way before. I still think graduate school is more stressful, though; I'm used to the stress of my family, it's been like that for many years. But I guess it may be contributing to why my panic symptoms started now.*

**Therapist**: *I'm not saying that's definitely what happened, but I think if we at least put that particular family immigration stressor on the table, we'll be able to look out for any thoughts that come up related to that when we start entering anxious situations or to better understand what state you might be in when your panic attacks occur. We don't need to talk about that one much more right now, and I just want you to know that if you want to raise the discussion about your immigration status or feelings about your family related to this again in the future, I am always happy to do so. It's just something for us to consider.*

*Summary of guideline application.* The therapist here is very skillful in balancing what may be related to a stressor for many immigrants in Tess's situation (uncertainty about one's status and emotions such as guilt related to those who have been left behind or parents who are still struggling as their immigrant children start to succeed) and still listening to the client about what she conceptualizes as the cause of her anxiety (the graduate school experience, which is very much a typical and broader stressor for many). Notice the therapist's empathy even when the client says the immigration-related stress is unrelated to her current symptoms, in terms of the supportive language he uses to let her know that it can still be discussed in therapy if she wants, on her terms. In this way, raising such cultural issues within the individual assessment paradigm is never wasted, as it continues to establish strong therapeutic alliance for the evidence-based therapy strategies that follow (such as exposure in this case). Similarly, the therapist is skillfully joining his expertise/observations as a therapist on how her overall stress level may be due to multiple sources (something that had not immediately occurred to Tess) with the client's own lived experience of being used to this immigration stressor and the new stressful context of graduate school. By finding this balance, the therapist can ensure that he does not simply assume that her symptoms are due to what may seem to an outsider to be more pressing (i.e., immigration uncertainty being much more "objectively" stressful than graduate school), thereby invalidating her reported experience.

## COMMON CHALLENGES

The challenges with finding the balance between culturally specific lines of inquiry and our standard interview prompts in the assessment process are unique because they include both our own personal barriers to engaging in this skill *and* also the institutional/clinic policies around doing so. Specifically, in terms of challenges that are less in one's individual control, your particular practice or training setting may not have the flexibility to add questions that get at more diversity-related influences on presenting symptoms if these deviate from their standardized battery of assessment instruments, because of time constraints in the intake process or due to lack of awareness of why such questions are important for adequate culturally responsive assessment practices. Such a program- or institutional-level resistance to incorporation of culturally informed assessments will be discussed in the "Putting It into Practice" section to provide some ideas of how to address this challenge (see also Box 3.2).

From a personal perspective, many of us have been indeed trained on semi-structured or standardized instruments (many of which do not include such

---

Box 3.2

COMMON CHALLENGES IN IMPLEMENTING GUIDELINE 3

* Less flexible policies in your practice setting to add questions that are not present on the standard battery
* Reliance on, or feeling more comfortable, using semi-structured assessment interviews that do not incorporate questions about identity-related impacts on presenting issues
* Uncertainty or discomfort around asking about identity issues, in terms of their relevance to presenting problems (**hint**: check out Box 3.1)
* Repeated assessment of the impact of identity-related factors on treatment goals and progress can feel forced or disruptive to clinical intervention/EBP focus.

---

culturally informed assessment questions as recommended here), and therefore we feel more comfortable staying within the limits of such assessments. This is very understandable; we all rely on what we have been taught and practiced the most, particularly if we have been in practice for a long time. As trainees, the idea of having to incorporate such questions without feeling that there is much structure to do so is a daunting task.

Further, even when we become committed to finding a way to incorporate such identity-based questions into our typical assessment approach, we can feel uncertain or uncomfortable about how we can actually do so in a way that is (1) respectful to the client, and (2) effective and useful for our main purpose of assessment, i.e., to determine the chief complaint and treatment plan. (If this is your main concern, Box 3.1 reminds us of some wording and prompts we can use.) Finally, both at the program/clinic level and personally, it can feel cumbersome to continuously assess for the impact of cultural variables or identity-related factors throughout the course of treatment, or even possibly disruptive to the EBP/clinical focus, particularly if the treatment approach we are utilizing does not have a standard inclusion of such issues in its weekly session and periodic assessment plan.

So how do we tackle all these very reasonable and yet addressable challenges in conducting culturally informed but person-specific assessment with our clients? The same answer for all our guidelines: practice, practice, and more practice! Let's discuss how, next.

## PUTTING IT INTO PRACTICE

Let's discuss how to tackle the barriers we may face in our quest to ensure we are engaging in culturally informed assessment at the structural level first. This is one of those places where we can be advocates and social justice proponents in our daily roles as psychologists. We can advocate with our supervisors, to clinic administrators, to whichever levels of hierarchy and decision-making authority we need to go to in order to ensure that questions that assess the impact of an intersection of cultural identities are being incorporated into the standard assessment practice. That sometimes means not taking "no" for an answer and garnering the support of colleagues and others in your setting in order to secure the approval and appreciation of its importance in ensuring equitable treatment of all those we treat, from the top down. I implore you here to rely on your own indices of privilege and power in your practice setting (whether that is conferred due to professional seniority or your own identity factors) to advocate for such a systemic change for your colleagues who may not hold as high privilege or power statuses in this service context (see Box 3.3).

On a personal level, it is worth the time to explore assessment batteries that more standardly incorporate identity facets/questions if you prefer to stick to something standardized or more structured, both in terms of clinician-administered and self-reported symptoms. Remember to check out Table 3.1 for some ideas for

Box 3.3

How Do I Practice Guideline 3?

1. **Advocate** with your supervisors, clinic administrators, or others in leadership positions of your practice/training setting to ensure that questions assessing for impact of clients' intersectional identities are incorporated into standard assessment practice.
2. **Explore** other culturally informed batteries you can become trained on or more familiar with that standardly include such questions (see Table 3.1) to supplement what you should also become comfortable asking in more unstructured ways (see step 3).
3. Become more comfortable through **role-play practice** where you ask these questions to peers, supervisors, or even in the mirror! Box 3.1 gives you some sample stems you can use to get more comfortable with the way to raise this line of inquiry in the context of assessment.
4. **Use standardized questionnaires** outside of sessions for repeated assessment for specific diversity-related factors (e.g., self-construal/cultural values, experiences of discrimination, acculturative stress; see Table 3.1 for some examples).
5. **Think of one question** you can periodically incorporate into your sessions to check in about the impact of cultural factors into your EBP; establishing this as an expected and acceptable line of inquiry in the initial sessions will help reduce the burden in doing so!

this, although this is certainly not an exhaustive list. Then, if you're still feeling uncomfortable or unsure about how to practically raise these issues in the context of assessment with an actual client, I encourage you to do some role-play practice using these standardized measures or some of the sample stems I provide in Box 3.1. Practice getting the words out with your peers, your supervisors, or even in front of the mirror. It will help make the wording more authentically yours and allow you to explore what internal feelings come up around talking about a salient identity factor in the context of assessment and treatment planning, particularly when those identity factors are very different from your own.

In terms of the burden that repeated questions around identity factors can put on the therapy process for repeated assessment/outcome monitoring, I would argue that as we become more comfortable periodically asking about such factors' influence on our treatment focus at hand, so that we are fully engaging in culturally responsive practices, this does not take much more time than other lines of inquiry that many of us are more comfortable with (e.g., assessing for the influence of our treatment on employment/school, family/intimate relationships, or reasons for noncompliance, and their reverse influence on treatment progress). However, one other way to reduce the burden of this additional line of assessment even further is to use standardized questionnaires related to diversity factors (e.g., cultural values, self-construal, experiences of discrimination, acculturation, or acculturative stress) along with symptom measures, several examples of which are provided in Table 3.1. By having these measures become a standard part of repeated assessment throughout treatment progress, this could inform changes that targeting presenting symptoms may be having beyond symptom reduction (providing possible additional areas of explicit discussion with clients) or possible barriers if treatment is not progressing the way you expect it to. Having such information over the course of treatment (even at just a few time-points) rather than just before and after treatment (pre–post) has the potential to greatly inform and improve the cultural responsiveness of your treatment.

Finally, let me return for a moment to my argument in the previous paragraph that we should each have even a brief way to assess for how identity-related factors may be at play over the course of therapy. If we raise this as an expected line of inquiry for our client from the first session, it will be easier to raise this again as we progress in therapy. Further, by asking explicitly about such factors and their relevance to the target areas at hand, we are signaling to our clients that they can feel comfortable raising these issues themselves in therapy, and importantly, that we view them as more than their disorder and rather, as individuals with dimensionality and layers to who they are as individuals. How can we not see that as anything but positive for establishing a strong working alliance with our clients? I encourage each of us to find that one question that feels authentically ours, where we can show this understanding of our clients as individuals who exist beyond their disorders and provide them with an acknowledgment of how unique factors may be at play in terms of buffering or exacerbating their presenting symptoms.

## COMMENTARY ON INCORPORATING SOCIAL JUSTICE

When we consider the main emphasis of this guideline, it really is about finding that balance between treating the client sitting in front of us as a unique individual, one who is more than their specific constellation of identities, and yet, whose identity/identities potentially greatly inform who they are and what they are presenting to us as their chief concerns in therapy. This is by no means an easy balance to strike, and we have to expect a fair number of instances of missing the mark by asking too much or too little about one's cultural background/beliefs (no matter how culturally competent we may think we are!). However, one core objective of social justice approaches within the field of mental health practice is ensuring equitable service provision, regardless of our clients' backgrounds. Thus, when we continue to practice finding this balance in culturally informed and individualized assessment of our clients, we are effectively putting in the effort to formulate the most equitable and tailored treatment plan and to address ongoing health disparities perpetuated from failures to do just that, at least one client at a time. Further, we can address persisting inequities in service delivery on a larger scale by advocating for broader sweeping adoption of such assessment practices (that include cultural/identity-based assessments for *all* clients, regardless of their visible identities) in our individual treatment settings. Finally, we are utilizing our own power and privilege in the role of the therapist to raise such issues that a client might be otherwise reticent to bring up, to empower them to bring all parts of themselves (that the client sees as relevant) to the treatment table.

## DISCUSSION QUESTIONS

1. What are some of the reactions you have to the thought of asking questions where you explicitly mention your clients' identity factors? If you have already tried doing so, what do you recall feeling while engaging in such a discussion? What did you find helpful and what did you find challenging?

2. How have you felt when others have pointed out your own identity factors (age, race, gender, nationality, or any of the broad identity factors that are most salient to you)? Did such a focus on your own identity generally bring up positive feelings, negative feelings, or a mix?

3. How might your own experience with having others talk about your identity, and how it relates to how you act or who you are, be influencing the predictions you have about how your client will feel about a similar conversation?

4. What are ways you have had others ask you about the salient aspects of your own identity that have felt welcoming and affirming? How might you modify or adapt those to be appropriate for prompts you can ask your own clients in the context of clinical assessment?

5. **Social Justice Action**: Have you received any resistance or pushback from supervisors or clinic administrators around the utility or relevance of asking clients about their intersectional identities? What are the ways in which you can start to tackle this resistance and advocate for incorporation of such questions (even starting small with one to two questions as part of the standard intake, to potentially exploring the use of a full culturally responsive diagnostic battery, depending on your practice setting's current policies) in order to ensure more culturally responsive and equitable assessment for all clients?

# 4

# Guideline 4

## *Engaging in Self-Education about Specific Cultural Norms Using a Variety of Sources*

## GUIDELINE 4 EXPLAINED

Even for those of us who have been already extensively approaching clinical work with cultural and diversity considerations in mind, it is impossible to know the nuances, cultural norms, expectations, and values that are central to each and every type of cultural or diverse identity group. Thus, continuous self-education about a client's specific salient identity factors (particularly if they relate to the problem at hand) is essential for maintaining cultural competency in clinical work (Asnaani & Hofmann, 2012). This effort is also closely related to the concept of cultural humility discussed in Chapter 2 (i.e., not assuming a perfect "state" of cultural competency and a reminder that this is an ongoing, career-long process). In addition, the sources of such education should vary to ensure adequate instruction on these cultural facets. In this way, we can obtain the most comprehensive view of how a client's identity impacts the psychological problem being targeted in treatment (Asnaani et al., 2022).

Such sources of information include (but are not limited to): (1) a review of the published literature on empirical findings about important cultural aspects we should consider in terms of treatment of specified problems in certain groups, or tested cultural adaptations to empirically supported treatments (ESTs) that may exist (e.g., Griner & Smith, 2006; Smith & Trimble, 2016); (2) working with the client to identify a trusted cultural steward in their community (e.g., a religious authority or community leader/advocate) who can be approached in partnership with the client to provide insight into important cultural considerations that may impact therapy targets and employed strategies (see Table 4.1; I also further demonstrate how this could look in our Case Application for this chapter below); and (3) consulting with colleagues with clinical expertise working with that particular community to obtain guidance on issues that may impede (or facilitate) a chosen EST for the client in question.

*A Cultural Humility and Social Justice Approach to Psychotherapy.* Anu Asnaani, Oxford University Press.
© Oxford University Press 2023. DOI: 10.1093/oso/9780197635971.003.0005

*Table 4.1* Local and Regional Cultural Consultation Resources

| Local | National/Regional | Networks/Repositories |
|---|---|---|
| Check website (or telephone) listings for locally based: | Look for mental health organizations specifically catering to the needs of distinct identity groups, such as:[1,2] | Check out written resources pooled together by clinicians and researchers working with a variety of diverse communities, such as:[1,2] |
| * Religious institutions<br>* Community social service or employment/ immigration agencies<br>* Cultural organizations (e.g., those putting together cultural events/fairs)<br>* State-level or city-level health disparities offices or community outreach teams<br>* Community mental health clinics located in neighborhoods with diverse clientele<br>* Language centers where various languages are taught | * National Alliance for Hispanic Health<br>* Indian Health Service (INS)<br>* Human Rights Campaign (HRC)<br>* National Deaf Center (NDC)<br>* Rural Health Information Hub | * Mental Health America (MHA) community-specific programs<br>* National Alliance for Mental Illness (NAMI), which has various community-specific pages/repositories<br>* Substance Abuse and Mental Health Services Administration (SAMHSA) Faith-Based and Community Initiatives |

Notes:

[1]This is NOT an exhaustive list! Find similar resources for any other specific identity group you wish to learn more about and rely on registered/recommended organizations versus individual/unverified resources online.

[2]Weblinks for these listed organizations are at the end of this book in the Appendix under "Resources".

As with our other guidelines, a first step here is to practice our self-reflection skills to assess whether we would benefit from additional consultation on specific cultural norms. (Note: the answer to whether you need to do this is almost always "yes," even if it's a cultural group you work closely with, because a brush-up on the latest literature is never a bad thing.) That said, this self-reflection can also reveal what specific sources of self-education are likely to be most helpful in your specific case. If you are unsure of the extent of your current knowledge base on a particular community or identity classification, look at Exercise 4.1 to do a self-assessment of what you might want to do to understand the relevant cultural nuances for a particular client.

Exercise 4.1

## Determining Whether and How to Engage in Self-Education about Specific Cultural Norms That May Be Influencing the Presenting Problem with a Client

After self-reflection on your knowledge and familiarity with the identity facets for your specific case in mind, start with the main stem question 1 below, and then review the recommendations for specific educational or scientific resources to use accordingly:

1. Are there salient parts of my client's identity that I definitively know are related to the presenting problems or treatment targets (either through assessment and/or explicit discussion with my client)? **If no, go to step 2. If yes, skip to steps 3–5. If you're unsure, review Chapter 3** on assessing for this more directly with your client, and then ask yourself this question again.

2. Even if upon assessment of identity-related factors you have a client who is not endorsing a connection of these factors to their target symptoms, it is not a bad idea to at least engage in **some initial review of major cultural rules/ norms** for the identity factor you guess to be most relevant to the presenting concerns (using your clinical intuition and conceptualization skills, ideally with some consultation/supervision). In this case, a review of the literature is at least warranted (look at the following **recommendation 3**, and only progress to subsequent steps if the identity factor becomes more saliently related to your therapeutic work or is revealed in repeated assessment to be connected to your therapeutic goals).

3. A first step across scenarios is **reviewing the empirical or published practice literature** on (ideally) the overlap between the specific cultural (and intersectional) identities of your client and how these have been studied in the specific disorder at hand, or if too narrow, then how these identities have been studied within the context of psychopathology/clinical psychology more broadly. Such a review will provide insight into the pooled knowledge (if any exists) for the clients we are working with, so we are not starting from scratch.

4. Next, **work with your client to identify someone** they ideally trust (and know personally, or can endorse as being a cultural authority in their current, local context) to be a representative of their particular cultural identity, i.e., a steward with whom you and the client would be comfortable talking to together (or you individually, if the client prefers) about how specific cultural norms overlay with the client's chief mental health symptoms. This individual will also be able to provide the therapist with important instruction on

specific cultural practices, beliefs, or challenges, so this burden does not fall on the client to "teach" the therapist about their identity factors. Further, such consultation with a cultural steward may provide better understanding about intersectional identity challenges your client may be facing, and will ideally provide better situational context about how your client's identities interact with the immediate societal environment.

5. **Share** with colleagues and supervisors about what you have learned in terms of the cultural norms and nuances at hand from both published and cultural steward sources to **obtain additional consultation and guidance** around whether your conceptualization about how these cultural norms overlay with treatment targets (and the treatment itself) is accurate, or whether you are still grappling with any crucial gaps in knowledge. Ask for suggestions for how such cultural values will need to be incorporated in your treatment plan (if applicable), particularly from colleagues and supervisors who have expertise in that specific cultural/identity group or have had their own extensive experience working with specific diverse populations.

While Exercise 4.1 has us engage in efforts that are certainly more time-intensive than our typical approach to case conceptualization and treatment planning, such an effort to access multiple sources of information on identity factors that have been raised by a client as being integrally connected to their presenting problems is important (Asnaani, Majeed, Kaur, & Gutierrez Chavez, 2022; Bernal, Jiménez-Chafey, & Domenech Rodríguez, 2009). Specifically, such self-education can conceivably help to reduce miscommunication in therapy, will strengthen the alliance and comfort level of the client with the therapist (particularly if there is a difference on a particular identity factor between both parties), and can set the tone for the overall structure of the therapy relationship (e.g., is your chosen EST going to be better received in a collaborative setup, or one that is more hierarchical or directive?). Further, remember that this process and integration of using various sources in one's clinical approach become easier with practice and will not be time-intensive forever! Let's see next how this might look like in practice in our Case Application for this guideline.


## CASE APPLICATION

*Case description.* For this guideline, let's return to our case of Rohan, whom we discussed in more detail in Guideline 1, where if you recall, the therapist was engaging in her own self-reflection about what she knew about Rohan's religious background (Sikh) and where she was less knowledgeable (including the ways in which this lack of knowledge was potentially fueling her own negative preconceptions of him as a person and how he may relate to her in therapy). As a reminder, Rohan is a 32-year-old, second-generation Sikh American, straight, cis-gendered male who lives with his family and works in his family business in an area which does not have a large Sikh community. His primary symptoms are consistent with a diagnosis of obsessive-compulsive disorder (OCD), and include significant self-grooming and other cleaning compulsions, along with secondary symptoms of social anxiety. Other notable features of his presentation and background include ongoing familial pressure to get married within his community, and reported experiences of racial and religious discrimination based on his adherence to important religious articles of clothing, such as wearing his turban.

*Evidence-based treatment approach.* Also, as we reviewed in Guideline 1 when this case was first introduced, the evidence-based treatment the therapist treating Rohan is utilizing is exposure and response prevention (E/RP; Foa, Yadin, & Lichner, 2012), which entails helping Rohan to gradually approach feared situations, thoughts, and objects that may bring on obsessions. Further, a key element of this treatment approach is to eliminate compulsions or ritualistic behaviors that maintain his anxiety, which is not going to be straightforward for this client given the entanglement of some of his cleaning/grooming compulsions with actual religious practices that are important to the client. Again, this treatment includes in vivo and imaginal exposure activities which engage clients in gradual approach of feared situations, thoughts, and objects that may bring on obsessions or avoidance responses that are typical in OCD. Treatment typically occurs once to twice a week for 60–90-minute sessions, with anywhere from 10 to 20 sessions to be considered a full "course" of E/RP.

*Preamble to therapy dialogue.* Following the steps defined in Exercise 4.1, the therapist first acknowledged both to herself and explicitly with her supervisor that (1) as noted above, her client's religious background as a Sikh was potentially central to the compulsions they wanted to target in therapy, and (2) that she was unfamiliar with the central tenets of Rohan's faith as a Sikh, along with some of the other cultural values related to gender roles and differences, with a personal bias that he may see her as inferior if individuals from his cultural and religious community regard women as subservient to men. It was clear from her self-reflection (as guided by her supervisor and the strategies outlined in Guideline 1) that she had several of these biases and deficits in knowledge around Rohan. She therefore first turned to the published empirical and academic literature to see if she could find information specifically outlining (a) the central beliefs and structure of Sikhism, including its organizing principles and origins; (b) any studies or published works on clinical considerations in psychology for clients presenting to treatment from this faith background broadly; (c) any studies specifically examining OCD treatment and E/RP; and (d) any published guidelines on incorporating and addressing faith-based beliefs more broadly into evidence-based treatments for OCD (e.g., work by scholars such as Rosmarin [2018]).

After engaging in such self-education on a range of related topics from reputable sources, she raised the issue with her client directly, with a clear rationale for how obtaining guidance from a trusted cultural steward or community/faith leader may be helpful for their shared treatment goals, as exemplified in the exchange below, which occurred early in treatment following psychoeducation around OCD and E/RP near the end of session 3 of individual therapy.

**Therapist**: *Rohan, as we progress with therapy and are starting to tackle some of the exposure activities we talked about today when we started making your exposure hierarchy, I think it will be important for both of us to get some guidance in the process. Specifically, you mentioned last week a few times when we put some of the items on your hierarchy that you weren't sure if they should go on there because some of the exposures could be directly counter to what your beliefs are as a Sikh and what is expected of you from your community. I assured you we would talk about those concerns after making an initial list, and I want to give time for that now. Can you tell me a little more about what was coming up for you with those items that made you concerned?*

**Rohan**: *Yeah, I'm glad you're bringing that back up, because it's been making me nervous. Like, I get how I need to stop doing some compulsions so that I am not anxiously thinking about getting dirty or being impure in some way, and a lot of that makes sense to me. But the parts we put down about not, like, cleaning my hair the way I'm supposed to might be directly in conflict in terms of what I'm supposed to do to show respect for the fact that I have long hair as a Sikh man, or don't do the things I'm expected to in terms of grooming my* beard correctly, for instance. I don't know if my parents or temple elders would think that's okay, and I don't want to disrespect my faith—it's important to me and who I am.

**Therapist**: *I totally get that, and I definitely don't want us to do something here that goes against your faith as a Sikh or feels disrespectful to that important part of your life. I have so appreciated what you have shared with me so far about Sikhism and what you find valuable and important about your faith. I want to also share openly that I didn't know very much about Sikhism before you and I started working together, and I have been working to read more about your faith and understand the important traditions, practices, and central parts of Sikhism. I still have a lot to learn, and while I have a better understanding now about the significance of not cutting your hair or removing facial hair, and that taking care of your hair is a sign of respect within Sikhism, I still can admit that I don't know all the particulars about what should be done and how/when. I also know that OCD often latches on to things that are really important to us, and given the fact that your faith is important to you, I am not surprised that some of your compulsions exist in that space. The tricky part will be for you and me to figure out what parts of your behaviors are in line with being a good Sikh, and which parts are your OCD. Do you sometimes struggle with figuring that out as well?*

**Rohan**: *Oh man, definitely. I often just assume that when there are cleaning or grooming compulsions related to my hair or clothing, particularly before I go to temple, that they are justified because they are what everyone in my faith does, and it sort of gives me an "out" in terms of resisting those behaviors or trying to change them. Wow. That's hard for me to admit, but it's true. I just feel like the stakes are higher, somehow, if I by mistake think it's OCD and then end up doing something offensive to my community.*

**Therapist**: *Very well said, Rohan, and I want to assure you that I don't think you're alone with that fear. It makes a lot of sense. What I find helpful in that case is to enlist the help of someone outside of our therapy relationship who can guide both you and me around what practices are expected and in line with religious practices and beliefs, and who may be able to provide an external (but trusted) perspective on what might be excessive. Often, we will call either a community leader or someone in the community who is knowledgeable about community or faith customs (not normally a family member, because they may be biased in other ways). Together, we will talk to that person and ask them to provide a blueprint for what the specific practices should look like (either from those they oversee in the community or their own experience), and then we use that as the anchor point for what parts of your own practice seem excessive so we can target the part of the behavior that seems compulsive, and not necessarily the whole thing. So, for instance, if that trusted person in the community says the average man spends X number of minutes combing his hair, or does so X number of times/day, then we would use that as our anchor and treat any urges to do so more than that guideline as part of your OCD instead of as part of good practices as a Sikh. Does that make sense?*

**Rohan**: *Ah, I see. That does make sense, and would make me feel better knowing that I am still doing what most folks are in the temple to care for myself in the way that is expected or respectful. It would definitely remove the pressure of me trying to make that decision!*

**Therapist**: *And for me, it would remove the concern that I may be asking you to do something that is counter to your core faith practices, which I certainly don't want to do! I'm glad you think that could be helpful; I have found this to be very helpful to have such guidance when working with clients of other faiths. Now who we chose as that "faith expert" can be very much up to your preference and comfort. It could be someone in your actual temple that you know well, someone in your temple you don't know well, or someone from another temple altogether (not even necessarily in our general area) who you think might be able to weigh in. Once we pick whom we are comfortable approaching about this, we can talk about what we are comfortable sharing about your OCD or not, and what specific guidelines we'd love to know about from the perspective of good practices within Sikhism. If you're open to it, let's chat about that now to figure out how to proceed so we can refine our exposure hierarchy accordingly.*

*Summary of guideline application.* The therapist provides a nice example of how to validate the importance of the client's faith or other diversity-related background practices and beliefs, while showing cultural humility in her own knowledge and areas in need of additional guidance. Notice how the therapist does not shy away from using faith-based words with Rohan (e.g., saying "Sikhism" and "temple" as the client uses them, instead of just "your faith" or "your place of worship"), which further aligns with her stated respect and desire to incorporate his specific faith into the treatment. She provides a rationale for bringing in an external person, and proactively provides different ways to do so that may address any hesitation Rohan has in bringing in someone he knows from his current place of worship (ranging from someone he knows well to less well to none at all). Once they establish whom they can approach and what specific questions related to his current compulsions they wish to obtain some guidelines or anchors around, she can bring this information and her own increased knowledge about typical practices and core tenets of Sikhism to her supervision meetings, as further advised in Exercise 4.1. Given her supervisor's own admission that she is also not very familiar with Sikhism, the therapist should be advised to seek out additional consultation, either through professional networks (asking if any colleagues have particular expertise around working in the OCD and Sikh community space, or mental health arena in this faith community more broadly) or enlisting the help of a colleague versed in the incorporation of religious values and practices into evidence-based practice, whom the supervisor can assist the therapist in finding (or one can use Table 4.1 to find themselves). Through this example, the therapist models the variety of sources which we have at our disposal and that we can utilize to better understand and meet the needs of our clients in the most culturally responsive manner.

## COMMON CHALLENGES

One of the biggest and most obvious challenges to seeking such a variety of sources to build our own cross-cultural knowledge relates to the fact that our published clinical practice guidelines and academic literature simply do not cover a very large gamut of cultural and identity groups, as this work is still in its relative infancy compared to other topic areas within our field (see Box 4.1). The additional complicating factor in this same vein is that our clients often present with multiple intersecting identities that influence the cultural norms or beliefs that we want to understand (e.g., there may be specific cultural norms governing female-identifying versus male-identifying individuals from a particular culture, or there is an intersection of considerations around one's age, sexual orientation, or gender identity and religious affiliation). Yet, our published literature is even less established in understanding such intersectionality in the clinical domain, making it challenging to obtain any insight or guidance around the identity issues that are most pressing in treatment. In these cases, relying more heavily on finding cultural stewards (as outlined in Exercise 4.1, step 4) would be indicated.

However, finding or utilizing cultural stewards/cultural experts comes with its own challenges. First, the client may not be open to the idea of bringing in someone they know from their community/identity background out of fear of being judged, misunderstood, or possibly suffering a loss of privacy about their mental health symptoms if the community is very small or tight-knit. Second, it may be that you are practicing in an area where your client is a particular minority

---

Box 4.1

COMMON CHALLENGES IN IMPLEMENTING GUIDELINE 4

* The client about whom you are trying to review the published literature is from a cultural group or intersection of identities that have not been yet studied or written about.
* Your client is not open to the idea of bringing in someone from the community who can weigh in on cultural norms and practices out of fear of being judged or having their privacy compromised.
* You practice in a place where there are no cultural experts or stewards in the community who you are able to consult with, or who are willing to talk to you.
* You do not know how to start even finding cultural experts or consultants for the issue at hand.
* You are not in a practice setting where you can consult with peers or supervisors about their identity-related knowledge.
* It feels difficult to seek diverse sources of information because your time is limited.

---

in that there are no established cultural stewards or community leaders with whom you can consult, or who are themselves not willing to speak with you as a mental health professional.

Luckily, the solution to both challenges is the same: you do not have to limit yourself to cultural experts who live in your immediate area/community, and in fact, you can seek out such feedback from such leaders who live elsewhere in the country to protect the client's confidentiality or to address a lack of such community resources where you practice. Then the question that arises as yet another challenge to engaging in such information-seeking and self-education is what happens when we are unsure of where to even find such cultural stewards (within or outside of our immediate localities)? This is not a minor logistical issue; fortunately, it is a challenge that many in our field face, particularly if we practice in more rural or culturally homogenous settings where we have a preponderance of a particular racial, religious, socioeconomic, or any other denomination of individuals. There are several resources that therapists can use in this case to find cultural stewards locally or nationally, as outlined in Table 4.1.

Similarly, Table 4.1 suggests resources for clinicians to consider around finding clinical guidance/consultation if you are in a setting where you don't have peers or supervisors who themselves have the experience or knowledge of working with certain identity groups. Compared to even a few decades ago, we have such a breadth of resources and knowledge available to us across our field (whether published yet or not), and relying on our broader professional networks allows us to tap into such cross-cultural knowledge and experience. Regularly relying on such networks is very much in line with good culturally responsive practice.

Finally, let's talk about time. Time is something that is already at high demand and low supply for many of us in the field. I am fully aware that asking you to engage in pursuit of a variety of information sources, as I suggest here in Guideline 4, is asking you to further deplete this precious resource of time. I would appeal to you, however, to think about how much of that same time will be saved by engaging in such varied and thorough self-education because it has the potential to ensure that your clinical treatment is effective, is relevant to your client, and is beneficial to your own perspectives on your own competency as a clinician. And very similar to our other skills, you will become more efficient and confident on how to refer to sources of information to augment your clinical conceptualization as you practice doing so and as it becomes more of a standard practice in your clinical repertoire.

## PUTTING IT INTO PRACTICE

So, here we are again—how exactly do we logistically put this into practice? What I mean is, Exercise 4.1 reminds us of the "what"—the types of strategies to practice this skill of self-education on cultural norms from a variety of sources—but *how* do we practically do it? This relates to the last challenge we raised in the previous section regarding limited time, and also has to do with timing of such efforts. This guideline dovetails nicely with the utilization of Guideline 3 (balancing cultural and individual considerations when assessing the client) whereby the adequate assessment of the client's salient identity factors early in treatment or during the intake will guide what literature you may want to review as your first line of inquiry, making this process of self-education more efficient and streamlined. This action also goes hand in hand with explicitly raising your intention to incorporate these identity-related factors into treatment with your client directly, and explaining clearly where you will be seeking information to educate yourself on the norms, values, and cultural rules that are important to that particular identity (see Box 4.2). Specifically, you want to make sure you assess for the client's comfort in bringing in a trusted/knowledgeable cultural steward or community leader into the therapy context to better understand the impact and influence of cultural factors in the work you will be doing together. You can give the client options about talking to such a cultural expert together or alone as the therapist (see this chapter's Case Application for ideas on how to raise this issue).

If the client is open to this discussion with someone they trust from their community, it is important to let them weigh in regarding whether they have a particular person in mind for such a conversation. If they are open to the conversation but do not have someone in mind or actively prefer not to have someone they personally know provide such guidance, you can rely on finding such a person from the sources outlined in Table 4.1, e.g., even regional or national chapters or branches of the particular identity group that do not have a direct connection to the client. If the client is not open to participating in such a conversation or is hesitant about bringing such a person in, you can provide reassurance that this is also a conversation you can have separately as the therapist to protect their confidentiality, and emphasize how such input has the potential to influence their treatment positively to ensure that the most holistic/comprehensive view is taken as you progress in your work together. If a client is still very resistant to such an idea, take a pause, and revisit the issue as you progress in treatment, particularly if the identity factors start to noticeably impact the effectiveness of your prescribed strategies.

Following a review of the literature and consultation with a cultural expert, remember to continue to consult with your colleagues about how you are planning to incorporate what you have learned in your treatment plan for the client's presenting issues (Box 4.2). If you do not have local colleagues who can provide such consultation because they also have had limited experience with incorporation of such sources of cultural information into ESTs, there are some resources at a national level that you can seek, particularly in terms of larger professional networks of providers or repositories of information (see Table 4.1) to obtain such consultation. While this step of information gathering is also ideal to do early in treatment with your client, it is equally important to have this be a periodic conversation and to rely on such consultation throughout the course of treatment, to ensure continuous self-education and application of your cross-cultural knowledge flexibly and responsively for the entire treatment duration.

Box 4.2

## How Do I Practice Guideline 4?

1. **Use your assessment** information where you applied Guideline 3 to understand the salient identity factors at play to start your initial review of published literature as your first line of inquiry. This should be done around the assessment session or before getting into the major treatment planning with your client.
2. **Talk to your client** in your initial treatment planning sessions about wanting to ensure that such identity-related factors (particularly if the client endorsed an influence of these on their target symptoms) are well considered by potentially eliciting the guidance or input from a cultural steward and/or cultural expert in the field.

**Ask**: *"How would you feel about us maybe speaking with someone about the norms or common beliefs from [XYZ identity factor] [or] in your [XYZ] community, just so I can fully understand what we would want to keep in mind as we progress in therapy? We can either do this together, or I can do this on my own, whatever you would prefer."*

3. If they are open to such a discussion, ask them about **whether they have someone in mind** that they would trust for you to have this conversation with, whether they will participate with you or not. Again, this should occur in the first few sessions of treatment during the planning stages. If they do not have someone in mind, then rely on the other sources mentioned in Table 4.1.
4. If the client is NOT open to participating or having such a conversation, **you can provide reassurance** that an alternative is to find a cultural steward outside of their immediate communities, or that you can speak to that expert alone. **Emphasize that getting such expert input** will make their treatment most effective.
5. After literature review and cultural leader consultation, **consult with colleagues** about the application of this cultural information to the clinical issue at hand, before and periodically throughout treatment.

---

## COMMENTARY ON INCORPORATING SOCIAL JUSTICE

Consideration of social justice within this guideline falls into two major domains, from my perspective: (1) improving our own cultural competency in order to provide more equitable, comprehensive care as therapists, and (2) empowering our clients to be part of the therapy process and be comfortable bringing parts of their own identities into their mental healthcare. For the first point, this benefit of Guideline 4 is quite consistent with the whole theme of this book. That is, when we take the time as providers to better understand our clients' backgrounds and improve our own knowledge about cultural nuances that are central to our clients' identities, we are working toward more culturally competent care, which itself aligns with efforts to address health disparities stemming from care that has ignored the impact of identity facets on mental health. For the second point, being transparent with our clients about our efforts to understand their backgrounds and our commitment to even bringing in cultural stewards and experts they trust into their treatment empower our clients to feel like their backgrounds matter, and they get a say in how such elements are incorporated into their treatment. Equity comes from sharing of power, which requires an acknowledgment that there is an inherent power imbalance between therapist and client which we are trying to mitigate. This guideline allows us to actually demonstrate partnership with our clients to shift this power dynamic into a positive, equalizing direction.

## DISCUSSION QUESTIONS

1. What are your own challenges to seeking diverse sources of information to inform your case conceptualization of a client? This can include external/ situational barriers, and your own internal barriers to seeking such information within the context of evidence-based practice (EBP) delivery.

2. Think about your own interactions with your own therapist, current/ previous supervisor, or in another professional setting: How have you felt when someone acknowledged the importance of an identity factor that is personally relevant or meaningful to you?

3. In that same scenario, how about when someone raises that without you raising it first, or focuses on it so much that the problem at hand is sidelined or minimized?

4. What do both types of experiences in questions 2 and 3 tell us about what we might want to consider when bringing in cultural expert opinion into the therapy room with our own clients?

5. What experiences have you had using one or more of the suggested methods of obtaining cultural input into your treatment with a client (e.g., reviewing the relevant literature, consulting with community stewards, or consulting with knowledgeable colleagues)? What was your experience with how well that worked, or the impact it had on your treatment delivery?

6. **Social Justice Action**: Think about how you can empower your clients (who are by nature in a vulnerable position due to a salient power differential with you as the therapist) to be an active part of the process of ensuring that all facets of their identity are given space in the context of treatment (if they wish that to be the case) by asking them to suggest a cultural steward to educate you as the therapist. **Don't burden your clients by having them be the primary source of education for you** by having them extensively explain all the values and cultural norms; as a therapist, take on that burden by doing the heavy lifting of seeking out information and just keep your client informed of your efforts, as this also implicitly shows them how important their identities are to you.

# 5

# Guideline 5

## *Addressing Stigma and Other Cultural Barriers to Psychological Treatment*

## GUIDELINE 5 EXPLAINED

As found in a number of studies, stigma around mental health and mental health treatment remains a major barrier to treatment-seeking, particularly for individuals who hail from specific cultural backgrounds (e.g., Eghaneyan & Murphy, 2019; Shea & Yeh, 2008). For instance, an individual identifying with a predominantly collectivist or interdependent cultural orientation may regard the need for therapy as a sign of weakness and source of embarrassment to one's family or community (Furukawa & Hunt, 2011). However, the influence of mental health–related stigma is not confined to just diverse cultural groups. Indeed, in keeping with a broader definition of diversity and the importance of intersectional identities, much has been reported in terms of elevated stigma toward mental health in certain age groups (e.g., older adults are more reticent to report mental health symptoms; Mackenzie, Heath, Vogel, & Chekay, 2019), socioeconomic status (e.g., lower SES is associated with a lower likelihood in seeking mental health services; Goodman, Smyth, & Banyard, 2010), religious affiliations (e.g., having emotional instability equates to spiritual deficiencies in some religious groups; Breland-Noble, Wong, Childers, Hankerson, & Sotomayor, 2015), and occupational roles (e.g., military settings where strong emotions are regarded as potentially dangerous and counter to the military culture; Barr, Davis, Diguiseppi, Keeling, & Castro, 2019).

Stigma has been posited to occur in three major forms: public stigma, referring to a perception that the greater community/society views the stigmatized group (in this case, those with mental health symptoms) as weaker or "less than" in some way; personal stigma, referring to an individual's own negative attitudes or beliefs about specific groups; and self-stigma, referring to one's internalization of negative attitudes or stereotypes toward oneself (Curcio & Corboy, 2020). These various types of stigma have been shown to influence individuals' attitudes toward

*A Cultural Humility and Social Justice Approach to Psychotherapy.* Anu Asnaani, Oxford University Press.
© Oxford University Press 2023. DOI: 10.1093/oso/9780197635971.003.0006

mental health and treatment-seeking behaviors. For instance, there has been a demonstrated effect of personal mental health stigma on the self-assessment of one's own mental health functioning and, subsequently, on one's openness to seeking treatment for mental health (Hahm et al., 2020). Further, public stigma has been shown to influence the broader public health system by impacting policy guidelines and funding allotments for individuals struggling with mental health issues. For instance, due to stigmatizing beliefs that mental health dysfunction is less important than physical health disorders, there are woefully deficient allocations in budget funding for mental health services in countries across the globe (less than 2% of the median health budgets worldwide; World Health Organization [WHO], 2017). In the context of therapy, then, and the mental health field more broadly, it is important to address the stigma around receiving such treatment with our clients directly, while balancing the provision of validation and respect for the client's perspective on mental health treatment based on their own identity backgrounds.

Aside from stigma, another cultural barrier that may impede the effectiveness of a therapeutic intervention in a therapy setting is the discrepancy that sometimes exists between the therapist and client on what constitutes an ideal working relationship between the two. Specifically, many treatment perspectives in Western contexts tend to emphasize a collaborative therapeutic relationship (Taber, Leibert, & Agaskar, 2011). However, individuals identifying with cultures that are hierarchy-based (e.g., South Asian or East Asian cultures) might expect a more directive, authoritarian approach in the therapy relationship (Chandra, Arora, Mehta, Asnaani, & Radhakrishnan, 2016), and thus, such a Socratic, open-ended style of questioning as typically utilized or valued in Western therapy contexts may actually end up raising doubts about the therapist's expertise and capabilities to treat the presenting problem in clients. Conversely, other cultural groups (e.g., Native Americans, or older European Americans; Hays, 2009) may regard overly direct questioning as utilized in certain therapeutic approaches as disrespectful.

Indeed, such a discrepancy in either direction between therapist and client on the ideal therapeutic relationship must be rectified and balanced; this does not mean that the therapist has to always be directive or can never ask questions in an open-ended way. The therapist also has their preferred therapeutic style that best suits their own therapy delivery, and instead, the style of communication and interaction might just have to be tempered to work within the client's expected treatment relationship framework. Again, an authentic and honest self-reflection by the therapist is important here, and it is perfectly reasonable for a therapist to work within the confines of how comfortable they feel with the level of collaborative versus directive interactions with their clients, based on their own training and perceptions of effectiveness. If there is simply not a match in this regard with clients, therapists who are aware of this potential barrier have an enhanced ability to make a determination of whether the client would be better served with a referral to someone who better matches their preferred style.

A third cultural barrier to actually engaging in psychological therapy with a therapist is a lack of trust in a therapist who is from a visibly different cultural, political, religious, or other identity factor from that of the client (Asnaani et al., 2022). Some of this concern has been traced back to a perception that a therapist from a different background will be less culturally competent in approaching the mental health issue at hand with the sensitivity, respect, and acknowledgment that is required, with evidence for a preference for providers who are already embedded or part of one's community (Gilmore & McAuliffe, 2013). More concerningly, some groups report significant concerns about encountering discriminatory maltreatment based on their racial (or other) identity from a therapist from a different identity (e.g., as has been reported in the Black community; Taylor & Kuo, 2019).

The issue of respect and adequate validation (particularly regarding how the client has experienced discrimination and microaggressions related to their various identity facets, and preventing perpetuation of such discrimination within therapy) is explored in the next chapter (Guideline 6). However, in terms of this concern around general cultural mismatch (and how this may impede implementation and reception of an evidence-based treatment), this barrier is not an insurmountable one. Rather, using texts such as this book to improve one's cultural competency and, importantly, the subsequent client perception of higher competency in their therapist due to use of the skills outlined here targets that very barrier. That said, this is another potential complicating factor that should be raised explicitly in the context of treatment, particularly if the therapist detects lower engagement or disclosure from the client.

Overall, Guideline 5 reminds us of these potential barriers to treatment engagement to underscore the importance of thorough initial assessment (and then periodic reassessment or explicit discussion) of an individual's cultural beliefs and influences (as we have discussed in Guidelines 3 and 4). This guideline also reminds us to consider the full intersection of identity factors and how these may influence engagement in therapy, to prevent ruptures in the therapeutic alliance and to reduce nonadherence to therapy recommendations. In the remainder of this chapter, we will look at how the therapist for one of our cases, Martino, detects some reticence and explores the presence of these potential barriers based on the therapist's conceptualization of what may be occurring within the therapy room and possibly impeding progress on the selected treatment protocol. We then examine the challenges to utilizing the tips exemplified in the case study and as suggested in Box 5.1 ("Sample Prompts to Explore and Address Potential Cultural Barriers to Therapy Engagement"), followed by ways to practice this skill with your own clients, and end with our social justice commentary on this guideline.

Box 5.1

SAMPLE PROMPTS TO EXPLORE AND ADDRESS POTENTIAL CULTURAL
BARRIERS TO THERAPY ENGAGEMENT

We explore some sample prompts to examine potential impact of the major cultural barriers discussed in this chapter; obviously, there may be other cultural barriers at play not covered here, and these prompts hopefully provide some model for how to address other barriers you detect as well.

### Stigma toward Mental Health and/or Treatment

* Normalizing stigma toward mental health/treatment: *I work with a number of clients who have shared with me that sometimes their friends, family members, or communities at large have some negative beliefs about mental health or going to therapy. Is that true for you? I would love to hear what some of those beliefs are so I can understand what that may look like in your unique case.*
* Using appropriate self-disclosure: *You know, I grew up in a household where mental health wasn't that valued or often not well understood. It took a lot of work for me to even try to understand why it might be important, and to do the work I do now. I wonder if you have experienced anything similar to me?*
* Setting up the stage to gently challenge stigmatizing beliefs: *You have spoken positively about how much your identity as someone from a rural Midwestern town means to you, and I know how important this part of your background is to you. What are some beliefs you hold in high regard or have positively influenced who you are today that you feel are connected to your upbringing in a rural, closely knit, small town?* [AFTER DISCUSSION]: *Have there been beliefs from this same part of your identity that you think are not the most helpful or important to you?* [AFTER DISCUSSION, IF MENTAL HEALTH BELIEFS DON'T ORGANICALLY ARISE]: *I'm curious, are any of the beliefs that have positively impacted you or that you don't see as relevant to what you value about yourself related to how you feel about mental health or even coming to therapy?* [GIVE SPACE TO DISCUSS WITHOUT FEELING YOU NEED TO DIRECTLY CHALLENGE AT FIRST].

### Discrepancies in Expectations for Ideal Therapeutic Relationship

* More directive line of questioning: *XXX, before we continue on our agenda for today, I wanted to ask you about how therapy is going. Specifically, how do you feel about how you and I are working together? Have you found my style of presenting information or leading us through the treatment skills to be helpful or unhelpful? Is there*

*anything I can do that would be more in line with what you were hoping I would be like when you were looking for a therapist?* [AFTER DISCUSSION]: *Thank you so much for sharing how you were kind of envisioning it, and those expectations make a lot of sense based on what we have discussed about your background in terms of* [BE SPECIFIC HERE IF YOU KNOW]. *I want to share a bit about how I think about therapy* [AS A PARTNERSHIP, A COACH, WHATEVER YOUR ORIENTATION IS].

* Less directive line of questioning: *XXX, before we continue on our agenda for today, I wanted to ask you a bit about what you think about therapy generally. What do you think a therapist is supposed to be like, and before you came here, what did you think therapy was going to look like?*

* Gently raising how a discrepancy may be impacting therapy: *So now that we have both shared what we think the ideal therapy relationship looks like, it seems like there are certainly some differences. I think it's very fair to think of a therapist as being someone who* [FILL IN SPECIFICS FROM WHAT CLIENT SHARED HERE], *and I get that looks different from my training to approach therapy as the therapist who* [FILL IN SPECIFICS FROM YOUR ORIENTATION HERE TO HIGHLIGHT ANY DISCREPANCY]. *I think one thing we both see similarly, however, is that we both want you to get the most out of therapy by* [STATE THERAPEUTIC GOALS WHETHER SYMPTOM REDUCTION OR IMPROVEMENT IN FUNCTIONING, ETC]. *To be able to achieve that shared goal, I wonder if we can find a way to reconcile or find a middle ground between the different ways you prefer a therapist to be and the way I am most used to providing care. Are you open to us coming up with a few ideas of how to find a compromise so we can help you get the most out of therapy?*

## Mistrust/Hesitation Working with a Therapist from a Different Identity Background

* Open-ended exploration of potential mistrust/hesitation: *XXX, before we continue on our agenda for today, I wanted to ask you about how therapy is going. Specifically, how comfortable are you feeling about working with me specifically as your therapist? I know it's never easy to talk about difficult things, but is there anything I can do to make you feel more comfortable or most safe to share what's going on for you?*

* Taking ownership/using self-disclosure: *I just wanted to make sure I asked this because I am very aware that I am* [NAME SALIENT POWER/ PRIVILEGE DIFFERENTIAL OR IDENTITY DIFFERENCE], *and that can make the therapy relationship already tricky, because it requires you to be more vulnerable with me. I am so appreciative for everything you share with me, and don't take anything you show the courage to share with me for granted or lightly. I know firsthand that when you feel really different or*

*vulnerable with someone else that it can be difficult to share everything going on. For instance, as a female in a primarily male-dominated science field, I often am concerned about being mistreated or that my opinions may be swept aside in professional settings where there are mostly men* [OR NAME ANY OF YOUR OWN AUTHENTIC POWER/PRIVILEGE/IDENTITY FACETS/RELEVANT SITUATIONS]. *Do you ever feel similarly hesitant to share anything with me either because I am your therapist, a woman, White, or grew up in the United States, or really, anything else about my identity?* [BE SPECIFIC HERE ABOUT HOW YOU DIFFER ACROSS INTERSECTIONAL FACETS, NOT ASSUMING ONE AREA OF DIFFERENCE].

* Showing commitment to the therapeutic alliance: *I want to make sure I do whatever I can to ensure that you get the most out of therapy, because I know it takes away your time and money to come here. I am committed to doing whatever I need to do as your therapist to make this a safe and open place where, even if we are different from each other in a number of ways or a few very important ones, you feel comfortable in sharing what you want to so you can get the most out of our work together.*

* Modeling how to brainstorm ways to address the mistrust: *I think it's very reasonable to be hesitant with me because I'm* [BE SPECIFIC HERE IF CLIENT PROVIDES THIS INFORMATION; DON'T ASSUME], *thank you so much for sharing that. I have a few ideas of how I can show you that you can trust me and hopefully this may help you feel more comfortable working with me, even if it takes some time, that's okay. For instance, we can make more space in our sessions for you to share anything you want to about how you have experienced other instances of discrimination based on your* [STATE SPECIFIC IDENTITY FACTOR HERE] *so we can better explore where this reasonable hesitation of yours comes from. I can also regularly check in about how I might be myself perpetuating some of this mistreatment based on your* [IDENTITY FACTOR], *to make sure I can check myself and immediately address anything I'm doing to make you feel hesitant about how much you can trust me. I am also happy to share some of my own experiences with how I have learned to build trust in vulnerable situations so you don't feel alone with having to do so. Another thing I am happy to do is to see if I have another client from a similar background who is willing to talk with you about how they felt working with me (without me being privy to that conversation) so you can get a more unbiased idea of whether I am a good fit for what you need, only if you and they are both comfortable doing so, of course. Do any of these feel like they may be helpful?*

## CASE APPLICATION

*Case description.* For this chapter and the next, we will work with our case study of Martino. Martino is a 62-year-old, Black, Spanish-English bilingual, cis-gendered male (nondisclosed sexual orientation) whose family immigrated from the Dominican Republic when he was a child and who was primarily raised in a major city on the East Coast. He was raised in a multigenerational house-hold, with the primary caretaker for him and his three younger siblings being his grandmother and one older sister. He had periods of time where he was with his parents, and observed domestic violence in the home, and significant alcohol abuse by his father (which often coincided with instances of physical violence directed at his mother and himself as he protected his younger siblings). At the age of 18, he opted to enlist in the military, initially to obtain financial support for college since his family struggled financially in mostly blue-collar and manual labor jobs (which also kept his parents away from home for long periods of time, resulting in his grandmother being his legal guardian), and per his report, "to make a better life for myself and get out of my [difficult] home environment." He ended up moving through the ranks of the military and doing well in his time there, being honorably discharged at the age of 42 after serving several tours in the Gulf War. He is presenting to treatment with symptoms that appear to be consistent with a dual diagnosis of post-traumatic stress disorder (PTSD), due to several race-based physical assaults perpetrated by his fellow soldiers, and alcohol dependence that started after these experiences upon his discharge.

*Evidence-based treatment approach.* Given Martino's chief symptoms (and the clinical conceptualization by the clinical team of his alcohol dependence being secondary and stemming from his PTSD symptoms), the primary therapeutic approach for this case is Prolonged Exposure for PTSD (PE; Foa, Hembree, Rothbaum, & Rauch, 2019). In this treatment, clients are provided psychoeducation on the common sequelae of having experienced a trauma (including problem-atic substance use), and then psychoeducation on the role that avoidance plays in maintaining recurrent, intrusive thoughts about trauma and other symptoms consistent with PTSD. They are then guided through the processes of in vivo ex-posure (via a jointly created hierarchy) starting in the second session, followed by the introduction to imaginal exposure (revisiting the traumatic event to pro-cess what occurred) in session 3. Exposure and subsequent emotional processing serve as the primary component of treatment for the entire course of PE, which consists of typically 8–15 sessions lasting 60–90 minutes weekly.

*Preamble to therapy dialogue.* Martino's therapist at the VA hospital setting where he is being seen is a 28-year-old cis-gendered male, straight, White post-doctoral fellow with considerable experience in treating PTSD and working with military populations within the VA system, where he completed much of his pre-doctoral practicum and internship training. PE has been progressing at a fair and protocol-consistent pace. However, the therapist is cognizant of the fact that he has not felt like he is truly able to "connect" with Martino, in that a lot of their

interactions are at the surface level, with minimal affect or sharing of details that
may bring up considerable affect as they engage in their trauma-focused work.

This reticence from the client at session 5 of PE is now starting to impede the extent of progress that the therapist and clinical team anticipated, and the therapist
has been advised by the team to consider what other factors are at play that may
be blocking the full engagement of Martino in therapy (in addition to the PTSD-
specific factor of avoidance, which is quite common for individuals who have experienced as difficult a trauma as Martino has). The therapist has discussed how
to approach potential identity-related barriers to engaging in the treatment with
his supervisor and peers, particularly in terms of not making the client feel like he
is to blame for the rate of progress, while still addressing these barriers to help the
client derive more benefit from PE. He now wants to raise these potential barriers
with Martino in session.

> **Therapist**: *Martino, before we get started today on our imaginal exposure and
> processing, I wanted to chat with you a bit more about how you're feeling about
> therapy more broadly. How do you feel therapy has been going, and what's been
> coming up for you having to come in to therapy every week, and having to do
> therapy homework at home?*

> **Martino**: *It's okay, I guess. I mean, I don't always understand why we have to
> talk so much about some things, but I know from our work here and my AA
> meetings that I have been running away from a lot of painful stuff, so I guess
> it's good to do.*

> **Therapist**: *I get that—as we have discussed, you have been so accustomed to
> not having to talk about certain things, and in a way, that was really adap-
> tive before when you were still serving so that you could get through your
> deployments. It's just less helpful now because the memories keep coming up
> and cause you to overuse alcohol, which I know has impacted a lot in your life.
> I think it's very reasonable to feel hesitant to talk about painful things that you
> have been avoiding for a long time, and you're not alone in doing so. Along
> with how recounting past difficult events can be challenging, I know that we
> each have our own beliefs overall about how useful therapy is, or what therapy
> should look like, or even how much is safe to share with a therapist whom you
> haven't known for very long. Maybe none of these apply to you, but do any of
> these additional things make it sometimes difficult for you to get what you want
> out of therapy?*

> **Martino**: *Hmmm, I guess in a way—why, do you think I'm not doing well in
> therapy?*

> **Therapist**: *Not at all—you're working so hard, and this is objectively hard work
> to do. I just want to make sure I am giving you the best possible service by pro-
> viding the space to talk about anything that either makes therapy harder to do
> or prevents you from getting the most out of the process, because I know how
> much effort you're putting in and it's not easy. I want to make sure I carry my*

*share of the load, and to do that, it can be helpful for me to understand other things that may be going on that make it harder to do all the things we have to—whether that is around beliefs about what it means to be going to therapy, preferences for what your interactions with a therapist should be like, or characteristics of the ideal therapist, or anything else.*

**Martino**: *Okay, I see. I mean, just coming to therapy is hard, like you said. In my family, nobody I know goes to therapy, and this was the thing only, like, rich White people do—no offense!*

**Therapist**: *Absolutely none taken, that makes a lot of sense. Are there any other messages from your family or other parts of your life that you have heard about therapy or mental health? I think these are all so important to acknowledge and verbalize given what we're doing here.*

**Martino**: *Yeah, I mean you know how it is in the military—only the weak need that help, though I'm glad to see that's changing a bit, there are a lot of young guys in my groups here, which I think is good. I never thought to go when I was younger and waited until things got really bad, now in my 60s. It just wasn't done, you put your head down and keep serving. There wasn't a place for me to be emotional or upset or whatever.*

**Therapist** [nods affirmatively]: *I can totally see that, and you're right, many of my clients here at the VA have said the same. So what I'm hearing, if I get this right, is that both in terms of your family beliefs and the military perspective, mental health is somewhat stigmatized or minimized, is that right? And I absolutely don't mean that as a criticism, but an observation about the way different groups in your life have regarded therapy. Does that feel like a fair characterization of what you shared?*

**Martino**: *I think so, yeah. And I mean, I find myself going back and forth with whether I agree with it or not. But I guess that does make it sometimes hard to take the homework or what we're doing here seriously. Like, is this stuff going to work for me, really? Or has it been designed to work for someone else?*

**Therapist**: *I'm so glad you're raising that, Martino—so insightful of you. And again, I think it's very reasonable to go back and forth in how much you think therapy will be helpful, because I'm sure there are a whole bunch of other beliefs you have been raised with or have adopted after your military time that are actually really helpful for you (like the importance of family that you have mentioned, or the value of hard work and persistence), so it totally makes sense to question whether this one might be in that category as well. I wonder if there are any other beliefs from your family or military service that you know off the bat are not helpful for you or have not served you well. How did you know those were not beliefs you wanted to adopt in your life or adhere to?*

**Martino**: *Well, things like if you aren't from the DR, you aren't part of the community—I learned growing up in New York that I had a lot in common* *even with my Cuban or Jamaican friends despite the cultural differences, so I have always been much more open to everyone than a lot of my family was. And also, I don't buy into all of this "America is the best" stuff that a lot of the guys I served with were into, even though I'm proud to be American. But those are clearly not in line with who I am—I think I am much more open-minded in general and think a lot of people have a lot to offer, no matter where they are from.*

**Therapist**: *Interesting! That is really fascinating to hear how two very different beliefs still kind of have this common element—you can more easily decide not to adopt them because they go against a core part of who you are and what you value about yourself, which is being an open-minded individual. That's great. I wonder, how does the belief that mental health is not so important or therapy may not work fit into that core part of you? Is coming to therapy and doing the work prescribed by it something that could be helpful for you, and is being open-minded about its potential (regardless of how it pans out) sort of in the same category? Or not? I'm not saying it is, I am just curious how you think about it so I can understand it better.*

*Summary of guideline application.* The therapist here is leading us through an interesting journey through detecting potential cultural barriers and addressing their role in the client's engagement in the evidence-based treatment. Specifically, you'll notice that the therapist starts off with a very broad line of questioning around anything that may be getting in the way, and then provides more specific examples of barriers (stigma, therapist interaction style, and trust in providers). The client, as someone who is bright and observant, immediately reacts with wondering if they are failing in some way at therapy. The therapist (anticipating this reaction) does a great job in ensuring that the client is not blamed or shamed for any perceived stall in progress. He shifts the focus on his desire to build his own competency as a therapist and knowledge about what the process of therapy is like for the client, and then reiterates examples of things that could interfere with therapy. He also validates the beliefs and explicitly states how much various cultural beliefs can be so helpful and powerful for the client's improvement and life in general. He offers a hypothesis of how this particular belief of negative perceptions of therapy might fit into other clearly rejected cultural beliefs for the client, without definitively placing it in that category. This allows Martino to think about how this particular belief serves him and intersects with what he values about himself as an individual, regardless of his family or military background. In this way, even if that's where the discussion is likely to end, this will permeate for the client as they continue with their agenda for the day. It will also possibly come up as a counterpoint in his mind when automatic thoughts about the utility of therapy arise outside of session, and potentially allow him to continue engaging in a value-based action of open-mindedness and hard work. Box 5.1 provides examples of the types of prompts you can use for the exploration and (gentle) challenging of cultural barriers to therapy engagement.

## COMMON CHALLENGES

It is interesting to talk about challenges here within a chapter that itself is focused on examining barriers, or challenges, to therapy engagement. But to be clear, here I want us to consider what *gets in the way* of addressing these barriers, "barriers to reducing these barriers," if you will. And this is a not a minor issue. For instance, before we can utilize the skills to address and reduce stigma that clients might have toward treatment-seeking that we discuss in our next section, what happens when the stigma level is so high that we can't even get clients into our clinical practice settings? Indeed, as mentioned earlier, the societal stigma toward mental health and its treatment services is a significant contributor to ongoing mental health disparities in diverse identity groups (Curcio & Corboy, 2020), which can be reflected in the (lack of) diversity of clientele you are able to attract into evidence-based practice (EBP). This is one of those areas in which our ability to advocate for minoritized populations and dedicate some of our professional service time to engaging with our communities becomes an essential skill for us to practice as mental health professionals. Partnering with broader organizations (such as your local chapter of National Alliance for Mental Illness [NAMI], or any other mental health advocacy groups in your area) to provide psychoeducation and community outreach on mental health symptoms and available services can address this stigma and even open up the possibility of treatment-seeking from those initially feeling too stigmatized to do so (see: https://www.nami.org). Such outreach can include providing service or educational flyers in cultural or religious centers of the community, offering a pro bono talk/presentation on a specific mental health topic of relevance to that community, or participating in ongoing health efforts (such as local community fairs) to bring awareness to mental health as part of a holistic view on health. Contributing to overall reduction in mental health stigma and literacy efforts in this regard are well in line with social justice principles and a way for each of us to individually address ongoing health disparities.

A second challenge to addressing cultural barriers to treatment is the fairly understudied possibility that therapists themselves may bring their own forms of stigma to the therapy relationship, based on our own internalized messages about mental health treatment, particularly if we identify with one or more salient identity factors that our client presents with in treatment. Self-reflection on our own biases and beliefs about mental health symptoms, as described in detail in Guideline 1, is crucial here, along with a practice of self-awareness of how these beliefs may influence interactions with clients (see Box 5.2).

Further, addressing cultural barriers such as differing perceptions between the client and therapist of what the ideal therapy relationship should be like (e.g., authoritative therapist-client relationship versus a collaborative partnership) can be complicated. Specifically, this is not simply a matter of orienting the client to a particular therapeutic orientation and its accompanying therapy style (such as a collaborative therapeutic relationship that is often prescribed by CBT). Instead, a client's belief that the therapist is an expert or authority whom the client does not

Box 5.2

## COMMON CHALLENGES IN IMPLEMENTING GUIDELINE 5

* Cultural barriers such as stigma or lack of trust in providers not from a client's identity group can stop individuals from even seeking treatment from you in the first place.
* Therapists bring their own forms of stigma to the therapy relationship, even if they match the client on one or more identity facets.
* Cultural barriers such as a discrepancy between how the client and therapist view the ideal therapy dynamic (e.g., authoritative vs. collaborative) is complicated and possibly linked to willingness to adhere to EBP.
* There is unwillingness by the client to actively address or discuss stigma; or difficulty in shifting client's beliefs that equate mental health with weakness.

question might be an important belief for the client to adhere to in order to have the confidence that treatment will work (i.e., positive expectancies) or to even engage in the EBP. Thus, the therapist will have to proceed with some appreciation for the flexibility they may have to show in their own preferred therapeutic style, particularly if the client seems uncomfortable with switching the dynamic between therapist and client away from what seems culturally congruent with their own expectations for therapy. This means that the therapist has to also be very clear on their own comfort level in modulating their level of authoritarianism and collaboration, and to understand these limits. If there is a clear mismatch, the onus falls on us as the mental health professionals to make a referral to another provider who is comfortable meeting the client at the therapeutic style level with which they are most comfortable to receive the EBP.

Finally, we discuss how to actively address stigma in the next section, but I wanted to preface this instruction by saying that even with our best efforts, some clients have strongly embedded cultural, societal, or familial beliefs that have equated mental health symptoms and/or treatment-seeking with weakness, deficiency, or inherent worthlessness in some way. And herein lies a challenge that can be viewed as one of those "tougher nuts to crack" in this sphere; how do we change beliefs that are both core to one's background/ upbringing and yet antithetical to facilitation of engagement in treatment or improvement in symptoms? I must admit, I do not have a sophisticated, evidence-based, or comprehensive solution to this. The best I can offer is a few of my own guiding professional principles to dealing with such cases: **persistence** in trying to adjust or gently challenge the helpfulness of such beliefs to that person's happiness and life goals, and **self-compassion** when I fail or fall short in that attempt.

## PUTTING IT INTO PRACTICE

The first step that precedes addressing potential cultural barriers to treatment engagement is, as always, assessment of such beliefs. That might include use of a self-reported stigma measure (e.g., measures such as the Stigma-9 Questionnaire or the Self-Stigma of Seeking Psychology Help; Gierk et al., 2018; Vogel et al., 2006), or reviewing the literature briefly for other measures that allow you to assess for potentially interfering cultural beliefs. You could make this a standard part of your assessment battery, as recommended in Guideline 3 (which is ideal), or you may decide to retroactively add such an assessment if you notice particular reticence or inhibition from a client during therapeutic exchanges (e.g., less engagement, limited responses/explanations of symptoms).

If you suspect that stigma, different expectations about the way a therapeutic relationship should be, mistrust of you as a therapist, or any other cultural barriers exist, we need to be explicit about it with our clients (see Box 5.3). To be clear,

---

Box 5.3

### How Do I Practice Guideline 5?

1. **Assess** for possible public, personal, and self-stigma toward mental health and treatment-seeking, particularly in a treatment-resistant or reticent client.
2. **Raise the issue** of stigma or other cultural barriers with client early in treatment (and periodically throughout treatment if needed as these barriers become salient); **explain** to the client that such issues can be obstacles to getting the most out of treatment.
3. **Explore** the root causes of the client's cultural beliefs; what messages did they receive from their families, communities, or society at large about mental health and what therapy should look like (including whom they can trust with mental health information)?
4. **Gently create some dissonance to these beliefs** by having the client reflect on the helpfulness of these beliefs, and raising some potential counterpoints to, or reframing of, some of these therapy-interfering beliefs, while still acknowledging how they are grounded in broader cultural/communal beliefs or preferences.
5. **Make a commitment** to client to keep checking in about how such cultural beliefs influence the work you're doing together (even if this means slowing down the pace of your EBP to ensure adequate engagement and buy-in) and ask them to take a curious, explorative approach about whether they notice any changes in these beliefs as therapy progresses.

---

this does not mean we are accusatory or blaming toward the client for a lack of treatment progress. Instead, (1) present the possibility of such concepts as being common for many clients, of many different backgrounds or identities; (2) describe what these barriers are and provide either observed examples or proposed suggestions about how they may be at play in your own therapy; and (3) explain why such beliefs may impede the client's ability to get better or get what they fully want out of treatment. Then, work with the client to have them self-reflect and expand on (as they are comfortable doing) the reasons why these beliefs or perceptions exist. Ask questions like, "*I have heard many different reasons why there is a belief that seeking mental health treatment means someone is weak or deficient in some way. I don't want to assume the reasons you may or may not have this belief; could you share a little about where this belief came about for you, in your life and your experience?*" Ensure that you ask several open-ended questions to make sure the client has a chance to fully explain why and how these beliefs are formed, how they see their impact on the treatment (i.e., whether they agree with you that such beliefs are impediments to treatment), and to get a sense of their openness to changing these beliefs.

Following this, it is time to gently challenge these beliefs and provide alternative views on the same belief as a counterpoint (without getting combative or into a debating mode!). For instance, as also shown in Box 5.1 and the Case Application with Martino, you can first validate the cultural congruence of the beliefs (e.g., "*I completely understand that in your community, you are not alone in feeling that mental health concerns are not as important as physical health concerns, and that's important for us to consider*"), and provide reassurance that you are not here to challenge core cultural beliefs or suggest that they are incorrect (e.g., "*I also know you are not alone in a number of other beliefs that are also shared with your community, such as the belief that elders should be respected and cared for as they age; I am not here to tell you which beliefs are correct and which are not, because they are all valid and consistent with your cultural beliefs*"). Instead, question the *helpfulness* of the beliefs, and do so gently and with an openness to resistance from the client (e.g., "*I do wonder, however, how you think the belief that you're weak in some way to come in for mental health treatment is helping you or serving you in having the type of life you and your loved ones want for you. I can see how respecting our elders ensures that your parents/grandparents feel loved and included and keeps your relationship with them close; how is the belief about being a weak person because you have been experiencing depression helping you in your life, your relationships, and with your depression symptoms themselves?*").

The last sort of tangible strategy that goes with this is an invitation to the client (whether they are immediately receptive or resistant to this initial line of inquiry into the utility of their therapy-interfering cultural beliefs) that this can be a conversation that you both explore together at multiple times in therapy. You can encourage a curious, explorative approach to seeing how these beliefs change (if at all), very similar to how we ask clients to take such an open approach to observing changes in their mental health symptoms over the course of an EBP. Doing so at least provides a way to revisit and continue to work over time, since many of these beliefs will not be reframed or loosened in just one conversation about them. Consequently, you might want to keep yourself open to slowing down the pace you typically follow in a chosen EBP in order to ensure adequate engagement in treatment and to make space for such conversations and any other suggested treatment modifications outlined in the literature that aim to make our EBPs more acceptable and culturally responsive.

## COMMENTARY ON INCORPORATING SOCIAL JUSTICE

Much of my work as a health disparities and treatment mechanisms researcher revolves around improving our understanding about why evidence-based treatments work better or worse for different communities and subgroups of people. To this end, better measuring and addressing the barriers that may impact engagement in evidence-based treatments becomes a key effort to increase access and uptake of such treatments across communities and demographic groups. By doing so, we contribute to reduction in individual mental health stigma (which may have trickle-down effects to the communities that clients are a part of as they share what they have learned in therapy), which itself is a way to address health disparities, as I mention earlier in the Challenges section. I also mention the potential utility of engaging in broader efforts around increasing mental health literacy in our communities, which further addresses ongoing health inequities, and could have ripple effects on improving uptake of effective treatments. Finally, one last point when thinking about increasing our advocacy efforts within our practice: as a health disparities researcher and a clinician who has worked with a number of diverse identity groups, I often encounter the fact that the very conceptualization of mental health greatly varies between communities (e.g., what is considered poor mental health?), and this itself may impede engagement in effective treatments. Such differences in conceptualization of mental health may be viewed as a barrier to the Western-centric evidence-based treatments and assessments we do, but it may not always be appropriate to try to challenge or change these. Rather, we can respect such differing conceptualizations from our diverse clients and work with them to figure out how to incorporate such beliefs into the treatment approach.

## DISCUSSION QUESTIONS

1. In this chapter, we have covered several distinct potential cultural barriers that can interfere with treatment engagement (including stigma, different preferences for the nature of the working relationship with one's therapist, or mistrust of a therapist), but what haven't we discussed yet? What other culturally based barriers have you observed that can interfere with treatment?

2. What are your own cultural beliefs related to stigma, ideal therapy structure, or anything else that may intersect with the client's beliefs or impede in the progress that the client can make in treatment with you?

3. What happens if the gentle challenging goes very poorly, and you recognize a clear rupture in the alliance by pushing on these core cultural beliefs? How can you utilize the skills learned in Chapter 2 (on cultural humility) to address this rupture and still stay the course of addressing these potential cultural barriers?

4. **Social Justice Action**: Think about your own cultural background and socialization into what therapy should look like. How much of this and your insistence on addressing this with a client (versus meeting them where they are at) is rooted in a Western-centric conceptualization of therapy? How can you come to terms with this bias, and raise it with peers/supervisors to ensure that you're adequately providing a space for your client and advocating for them to bring their own culturally congruent beliefs into EBP? How about when you notice it with others in your group supervision/training sessions, i.e., what can you do to advocate for others' clients?

# 6

# Guideline 6

## *Exploring the Impact of Discrimination and Microaggressions on Therapy*

## GUIDELINE 6 EXPLAINED

When I first started teaching about practical ways to be culturally competent within the context of delivering evidence-based treatments, I often recommended giving clients the space to share their individual life stories if they wish to do this, in line with culturally competent practice (Coronado & Peake, 1992). I would add experiences of identity-based discrimination and oppression as examples (among others) of some of these life experiences. However, as my thinking about the importance of these variables and my own multifaceted identity have evolved over the course of my clinical and research career, I realize just how much I have missed the mark in my previous teaching in this area. What I mean to say is that I am now much more emphatic that we absolutely must provide such a space, specifically and explicitly, for clients to share how they have experienced racism, sexism, ableism, homophobia, and any other slew of unfair and unfortunate treatment based on their specific (and often intersectional) identity factors. Further, we should be proactive in our validation of, and willingness to discuss, these experiences (Kelly, 2006; Vasquez, 2007). Part of culturally humble and socially just practice is provision of a consistently dedicated space to discuss the experience of both overt discrimination and microaggressions (which, despite the use of the descriptor "micro," are still extremely impactful and perhaps better captured by the contemporary term "identity-based aggression"; Pinder-Amaker & Wadsworth, 2022).

Indeed, we can effectively engage our clients in this often-difficult conversation around past experiences of overt and covert discrimination (broadly, and perhaps as they have experienced within the context of therapy) with several key strategies in mind (see Table 6.1). First, provide validation and empathy around the client's prior experience—this is a key time to build alliance and show positive regard for your client's lived experience, as this will assist in reducing the client's

*A Cultural Humility and Social Justice Approach to Psychotherapy.* Anu Asnaani, Oxford University Press.
© Oxford University Press 2023. DOI: 10.1093/oso/9780197635971.003.0007

*Table 6.1* WHAT TO DO WHEN YOUR CLIENT RAISES EXPERIENCES OF PREVIOUS DISCRIMINATION IN THERAPY

| Validate and empathize with their experience | In the initial report, **let the client lead** the level of detail and feelings they want to share about their experience | **Express a commitment** to doing your best to ensure you don't discriminate or perform microaggressions as a therapist |
| --- | --- | --- |
| <u>Try</u>: "I'm so sorry you had to experience that. That must have been so difficult, and I am so glad you brought it up here." | <u>Try</u>: "I'm here to listen to anything you want to share about that experience, in terms of what happened and/or what you felt. There is no pressure to share more than you feel comfortable doing." | <u>Try</u>: "I definitely want this to be a place where you feel safe, not judged and one where you feel completely valued for who you are. I will work hard to make sure I do everything I need to for our therapy to be that place for you. I will always be open to hearing if you ever feel like it's not so I can correct what I need to in my behavior to make sure it is." |
| <u>AVOID</u>: "Are you sure that really is what that person meant? Could it be that they didn't mean anything discriminatory?" | <u>AVOID</u>: "Can you tell me exactly what was said or what happened next? Tell me more about how that made you feel and let's break down what happened for everyone involved." | <u>AVOID</u>: "Please make sure you explain to me or tell me when I might be committing a microaggression. I won't be able to tell I'm doing so unless you let me know, so please make sure you do." |

hesitation around discussing such issues as therapy progresses (Vasquez, 2007). There should be no qualifiers or excuses in the way you provide this validation (e.g., avoid using wording like "*I can see how you might view that as discriminatory*" and instead consider "*I am so sorry you experienced such a difficult or discriminatory experience*").

Relatedly, consider that while it may be tempting to get as much detail as you can about what happened and how the client felt (and how these reported experiences may be related to their current presenting problem), this may not be the ideal way to process such experiences. For instance, I have noticed in my own work (and experienced firsthand) that talking about experiences of discrimination can be very painful for individuals and can exhaust much of one's emotional capacity. Particularly in initial discussions about these experiences, clients should be allowed to share as much or as little as they wish about these experiences, and this is not the time to probe for more detail than they feel comfortable sharing. When clients first raise such experiences, they want to feel believed and receive support; this should be the sole focus initially, and clinicians should only later examine how much that experience has influenced the current symptoms as the alliance strengthens with the client (Kelly, 2006).

Finally, regardless of how much clients share about their experiences of unfair and harmful treatment in general or previous therapy contexts, one additional way that you can create a safe space for your client to continue sharing such experiences is to explicitly state your commitment to working on what you need to as the therapist to make the therapy space one that is free from such biased treatment. This could be a powerful statement that could facilitate your client feeling more comfortable raising any discriminatory or microaggressive treatment they have experienced. In addition, such a statement can give clients the reassurance that they can safely elaborate on other experiences that they have been reticent to share, and that you will provide a nonjudgmental, open space for them to do so.

In fact, this last point of creating a space where clients can safely raise issues of discrimination is particularly important, given that microaggressions can very possibly occur *within* the context of therapy and *may be perpetuated by ourselves as the therapist* (Lee, Tsang, Bogo, Johnstone, & Herschman, 2018), as we saw in our case example in Chapter 2 (guideline on cultural humility) and as alluded to in the final column of Table 6.1. As reviewed in the Introduction, microaggressions can be conceptualized as falling squarely under the umbrella of discrimination, in that they point us to the ways in which individuals can experience what might seem as minor/commonplace intentional or subconscious insults based on one's identity markers, but that have cumulative and individual deleterious impacts on those receiving such microaggressions (Nadal et al., 2015). For instance, several studies have implicated the experience of microaggressions and discrimination in poorer mental and physical health outcomes (Carter, Lau, Johnson, & Kirkinis, 2017; Chou, Asnaani & Hofmann, 2012), and these experiences can occur in the context of specific and separate identity markers (e.g., based on one's gender identity, such as being misgendered), or in intersectional identity terms (e.g., the harmful trope of the "angry Black man"). The incidence of microaggressions occurring because of dynamics within the therapeutic relationship, on the other hand, is fairly less examined and is only now growing in its examination (Nadal et al., 2015; Owen et al., 2018).

For instance, several studies have shown that microaggressions as perpetuated by the therapist are experienced in roughly 50% of clients identifying as ethnic or racial minorities (Owen, Tao, Imel, Wampold, & Rodolfa, 2014), and clients of other diverse identity backgrounds based on gender identity, sexual orientation, religion, or disability status have also reported the experience of such therapist-perpetuated microaggressions (Nadal et al., 2015; Shelton & Delgado-Romero, 2011). This research has further revealed that therapists are often unaware that they have committed such microaggressions, or more frequently, might opt not to address the rupture in alliance that often occurs as a result. Choosing to ignore such microaggressions/missteps comes at a cost: studies show that those therapists who exemplify their cultural humility and potential missteps with clients are more likely to reduce the frequency of such microaggressions and dampen their impact on clients than those who choose to ignore or not raise what happened in therapy with their clients in a culturally humble manner (Hook, Davis, Owen, Worthington, & Utsey, 2013).

Certainly, the data are clear that our best course of action in the case of discrimination and microaggressions is not to commit such offenses to begin with, given the extensive potential detrimental effects on our clients' well-being. We cover what to do when we actually commit a microaggression (as one potent form of a cultural misstep) in Chapter 2, but what about those who say, it's all fine and well to have steps to repair a rupture due to a microaggression I inadvertently perform in therapy, but what if I'm not even aware that I committed one? That is a great question, and another skill we must develop that is closely related to this guideline in our quest to be culturally responsive therapists. Box 6.1 guides us through ways we can ensure preventatively that we do not perpetrate such microaggressions with our clients. For instance, we are reminded here of the importance of consistent and repeated self-reflection about our own biases and discriminatory experiences. Some ways to make our own biases more salient is through private self-reflection, discussion with trusted peers and supervisors, being mindful in the session about negative reactions and thoughts to identity markers of our clients, reviewing sessions to observe nonverbal biased behaviors toward our clients, or completing implicit bias tests or one of the numerous exercises developed by colleagues to

---

Box 6.1

## How Can I Be Mindful about NOT Committing Microaggressions in Therapy?

* Engage in self-reflection about your own current biases as we cover in Guideline 1 (remember: this is continuous process throughout your career!).
* Discuss these potential areas of judgment/bias with supervisors and peers to generate ways for you to address them outside of your time with your client.
* During sessions with clients, notice your negative reactions and thoughts to their salient identity markers; if in-the-moment awareness is difficult for you, reflect and write about how you felt in the session or watch videos/listen to sessions to see if you can more objectively view your body language/verbal expressions that may be related to your own biases.
* If there are still gaps in our knowledge about where our own biases may lie, consider engaging in implicit bias tests or other exercises that help us tap into such biases that may be at play outside of conscious awareness (see end of this chapter and text resources for more on this).

---

become more aware of our own performed microaggressions and biased beliefs (e.g., Togans, Robinson, & Meredith, 2014; www.breakingprejudice.org at Ball State University).

There are two other areas that are pertinent to understanding the impact of microaggressions within the therapeutic context. One occurs when therapists are on the receiving end of microaggressions from either clients or their own supervisors; I cover this in detail in Chapter 9 on considerations for supervision. The second is when we notice microaggressions being directed to our clients by others on the clinical team (whether or not this is done in the client's presence) or within a group treatment context by other members of the group. While the most effective strategies for addressing such microaggressions occurring in the therapeutic context are still being empirically examined, initial studies have shown support for several clear corrective steps. Derald Wing Sue and colleagues have provided considerable and sage guidance detailing these strategies, along with other experts in the cultural competency field (Lee et al., 2018; Sue et al., 2007; Sue et al., 2019). Some of these guiding steps have been already covered in Chapter 2 when we discussed addressing cultural missteps when we are the perpetrators of microaggressions, but here we review the specific steps for addressing microaggressions and blatant discrimination perpetrated by others when they occur within the context of therapy, which our Case Application for this chapter will also demonstrate.

Specifically, Sue and colleagues encourage us to think about the ways we address microaggressions using any of these approaches as "microinterventions" (Sue et al., 2019). First, Sue and colleagues advise us that we need to be explicit about the microaggression that has occurred, and "make the invisible visible," so that we are very clear about the specific violation that has occurred (either by ourselves, as I exemplified in Chapter 2, or when we observe it being perpetrated by others). Second, if you're observing the microaggression occurring as perpetuated by someone else, instantly call out the microaggression as something that you disagree with or disapprove of to disarm its impact and to stop it in its tracks. This can be coupled with actively serving as an ally by providing education to the offending individual about why such a statement or action is prejudicial or discriminatory. Another microintervention that can be used in conjunction with any of these is to obtain support from your practice setting at large, and external reinforcement for a climate of inclusion and equity, with statements released from the administration at large that any discriminatory behavior will not be tolerated, or from peers who can provide allyship as well. Exercise 6.1 provides a way to reflect on such observed microaggressions and to figure out what steps from these and other suggested strategies may be most called for in the situation at hand. Remember: regardless of our own individual identity factors, we hold power and privilege in the therapy relationship with our clients, and being an ally for them (whether they are aware of it or not) is a way for us to practice being socially just, ethical, and equitable therapists who are committed to ensuring fair treatment for all.

Exercise 6.1

ADDRESSING MICROAGGRESSIONS WHEN WE OBSERVE OTHERS IN OUR
PROFESSIONAL SETTINGS COMMITTING THEM TOWARD OUR CLIENTS

**1. Reflect here on what specifically happened that you believe was a microaggression directed toward your or another's client.**

What specifically happened? What was the microinsult/microassault that occurred, and who was the target and the perpetrator?

Nature of microaggression: _____

Perpetrator (identity, role, etc.):_____

Target (identity, role, etc.):_____

**2. When this incident occurred, what did you feel? What thoughts came up, and did you have an immediate or delayed recognition that a microaggression had occurred?**

_____

_____

**3. When this incident occurred, how did others (if applicable) react or respond?**

_____

_____

**4. What can you say to practice naming the specific microaggression that occurred explicitly?**

_____

_____

_____

* If you didn't say this when it occurred, and you're reflecting on this after the incident has already occurred, when can you next state what you came up with above with the offending individual?

_____

**5. What language can you use that is appropriate within that setting (whether it's within a clinical team meeting versus a group treatment session and your target is a colleague versus another client) to express your clear disapproval of the microaggression to disarm it?**

_____

_____

_____

**6. What kind of education might be most effective to provide to the offender to explain why their words or actions were microaggressive? List a few points you could refer to here.**

Point 1: _____

Point 2: _____

Point 3: _____

**7. Who can you approach in your clinical team, organization, or administration to share what happened and obtain more institutional/broader support around this incident to ensure it is addressed more fully by your practice setting?**

Colleagues: _____

Supervisors: _____

Administrators: _____

External scholars/Networks: _____

_____

To see how engaging in such strategies and reflection in Exercise 6.1 might look like in action, let's consider the following situation that unfolded with our case Martino, whereby the client's therapist observed the microaggression occurring within the context of a clinical team meeting. The first dialogue provides an example of what occurs when the therapist chose not to address it, followed by a second dialogue modeling the therapist actively addressing the observed microaggression.

## CASE APPLICATION

*Case description.* As we discussed in the previous chapter, Martino is 62-year-old, Black, Spanish-English bilingual, cis-gendered, male veteran (of undisclosed sexual orientation) presenting with symptoms of post-traumatic stress disorder (PTSD) and alcohol dependence, and our therapist treating him is a 28-year-old, cis-gendered male, straight, White postdoctoral fellow. Martino was raised in a multigenerational household, with the primary caretaker for him and his three younger siblings being his grandmother and one older sister. At the age of 18, he opted to enlist in the military, initially to obtain financial support for college since his family struggled financially in mostly blue-collar and manual labor jobs and, per his report, "to make a better life for myself and get out of my [difficult] home environment." He ended up moving through the ranks of the military and doing well in his time there, being honorably discharged at the age of 42 after serving several tours in the Gulf War. He is presenting to treatment with co-occurring diagnoses of PTSD and alcohol dependence, which have impeded his ability to hold down civilian employment as a result. Of note, Martino reported that he uses alcohol on a consistent basis to mask distressing memories about several distinct events that occurred during his time serving in the military, two notable ones of which occurred when he was just starting his service, and were related to racial discrimination and physical violence perpetrated by his fellow comrades.

*Evidence-based treatment approach.* Also, as we reviewed in the previous guideline (Chapter/Guideline 5) when this case was first introduced, the evidence-based treatment of choice for Martino was deemed to be Prolonged Exposure (PE; Foa, Hembree, Rothbaum, & Rauch, 2019), which entails psychoeducation on commonly occurring symptoms of PTSD and co-occurring symptoms (such as alcohol dependence, the other central piece of Martino's clinical presentation), and then a focus on the gradual approach of situations, people, and activities that the client has been avoiding (in vivo exposure) or thoughts/memories of a trauma (imaginal exposure) over 8–15 weekly sessions. In the previous chapter, we observed a conversation between Martino and his therapist around some of the barriers he is experiencing in terms of engaging in PE (e.g., beliefs about the utility of therapy, stigma toward mental health, and concerns about the generalizability of effectiveness of PE with diverse cultural groups).

*Preamble to therapy dialogue.* In this current excerpt from Martino's treatment, the therapist was providing information about what had occurred in his latest session with Martino during a clinical team meeting in which his supervisor (a White, early-career female), other postdoctoral fellows and several practicum students (representing a range of identities), and several other licensed clinicians on the team (a Black advanced-career male, a Latina early-career female, and a White advanced-career female) were present. The therapist was describing Martino's reticence about engaging in therapy based on his cultural and military background (as we explored in Chapter 6 on stigma), and he was about to describe how he skillfully assessed for and addressed this cultural barrier that was perhaps impeding in treatment for Martino's PTSD. However, before getting into this part of his retrospective account of what occurred in therapy, a microaggression occurs, perpetrated by the White advanced (senior) female licensed colleague (not his supervisor).

**Therapist** [just finished recounting what he learned from Martino about his perspective on therapy and how this is influenced by family/military culture per the client dialogue in the previous chapter]: *So, with this information in mind, I now have a better sense of why Martino seemed a bit less engaged or forthcoming with how he feels in therapy. I think knowing this can really help us in moving forward—*

**Offending clinical team member** [interrupting]: *I mean, sort of, right? Being hesitant to come to therapy is pretty typical of most people of color. Part of it is that these communities aren't very educated and don't know much about mental health, so it makes sense they are hesitant to come in. Also, this work is hard, so it's easier to just not engage for some people. I don't think your client shared anything we don't already know about his community and I don't know how much we have to take this into account in trying to get him to just engage in PE.*

**Therapist**: *Well, I guess we know that stigma about mental health is a big deterrent to coming into therapy, yes. But I think that in Martino's case specifically, it might be useful to think about how his concerns about therapy are multifaceted based on both his cultural background and also his long-standing military background. What I then did to see if we can address the issue was to . . .* [goes into description of what he did to address this potential barrier to treatment engagement as described in the previous chapter, choosing to disregard the microaggression that occurred].

In this scenario, the therapist, even if he notices the multiple microaggressions and microinsults performed by the senior member of the team, chooses to minimize or deflect this violation and focus on what he did as a therapist to shift attention back to the clinical issue at hand. Nevertheless, he is likely quite aware (as many in the room are) that a microaggression has occurred toward his client and he is probably grappling with some shame, embarrassment, anger, and confusion about how to address it when he is not the perpetrator. Undoubtedly, many of us have been in a similar situation: Do we call out clear bigotry at the expense of our own careers and training, particularly when a power differential exists within supervisory situations? How do we do so without seeming offensive, accusatory, or "oversensitive" ourselves? What responsibility do we have to call out offensive behavior from those more senior than us when there are other senior individuals who are also witnessing such behavior? Many such thoughts likely occurred very quickly for this therapist in terms of how he should respond in a way that balances addressing what Martino needs clinically and yet what is the socially just thing to do to address the treatment the client is receiving, even though the client is not in the room. Further, the dynamics of the situation (multiple trainees and supervisors/licensed clinicians who are themselves of varying expertise and minority backgrounds) likely makes it more complicated for this therapist, and is not an unusual setup for many clinical settings. Now let's take the same situation and see what would happen if the therapist, despite these team power dynamics, adopted the recommended approach outlined above of proactively and explicitly addressing the microaggression and acting as an ally to their client.

**Offending clinical team member** [interrupting]: *I mean, sort of, right? Being hesitant to come to therapy is pretty typical of most people of color. Part of it is that these communities aren't very educated and don't know much about mental health, so it makes sense they are hesitant to come in. Also, this work is hard, so it's easier to just not engage for some people. I don't think your client shared anything we don't already know about his community and I don't know how much we have to take this into account in trying to get him to just engage in PE.*

**Therapist**: *I think that's unfair to assume, actually, Dr. X. First, by reducing Martino to just one part of his identity (in this case his racial and cultural identity) does him a disservice because he is made up of an intersectional set of experiences and identity facets. For instance, he made it clear that it was a combination of his family beliefs and military background that led to particular reticence. Further, I do think we need to be mindful as a team to not use language that belittles or insults the education level of whole groups of individuals— maybe that was not your intention, but that's what I heard. I think this sort of labeling or "othering" of specific communities is problematic, and undercuts the kind of clinical services we can provide to our clients when we are dismissive of who they are and what specific and unique cultural factors are at play that may be interfering with treatment engagement.*

**Offending clinical team member** [visibly getting angered]: *Okay, okay, just hang on, let's not make this a whole race thing. You know that's not what I meant, and also, it's common knowledge that people who come from where he comes from don't really believe in mental health, and tend to come here with not a lot of education in general. So I didn't say anything that isn't correct.*

**Therapist**: *Again, I respectfully disagree. I think we can work with basic tenets of understanding about how groups of people generally think about mental* *health, but I think we can still do so in a way that is not dismissive or insulting to entire groups of people. For instance, I found your characterization that therapy is hard work and that it is easier to just not engage for "some people" in the same breath as referring to Martino's Hispanic and immigrant background. Even right now, you referred to "people who come from where he comes from," which I think continues to other him as a client, which, again, I know is not likely your main intention. Yet, such statements take away from us understanding as a clinical team how his specific family beliefs, which are rooted in both Dominican Republic but also American values, and which intersect with other parts of his identity, may be influencing what I see, frankly, as valid reticence to engage in therapy. Language, regardless of intention, matters, and I have learned that firsthand. I'd like to hear what other members of the team think about my concern about why we need to work hard as a team to refer to our clients in the most respectful and open-minded ways, and whether your assessment was received as negatively as I did before we continue discussing the clinical issue at hand.*

Author note about this exchange above: I'm often asked by colleagues who want to be allies and yet, understandably, feel very hesitant to do so and be perceived as "oversensitive" or offensively politically correct while doing so, about how to proceed when they witness the many microaggressions we each have unfortunately witnessed, as described above. My answer? If you found the above exchange difficult to read and feel like you couldn't possibly envision yourself saying what this therapist had the strength to do, imagine how your client would have felt to be addressed as "those people" or reduced to a specific identity factor (or hear his loved ones characterized in such ways). Our discomfort and feelings of awkwardness, quite honestly, pale in comparison to what individuals who are on the receiving end of microaggressions have to deal with in so many situations throughout their lives. I implore you to dig deep into your own well of strength and resilience to be that advocate for your clients.

*Summary of guideline application.* Thus, when being socially just, culturally competent therapists, we make the commitment to do what this therapist did: (1) call out what specific microaggression occurred; (2) highlight how this undermines effective treatment of diverse (and all!) clients; (3) point out how such behaviors impact other members of the team, particularly if they are also of minoritized backgrounds, though I would argue just in general as well; and (4) elicit commitment and support from other members of the team to combat such mistreatment so that we can stamp such microaggressive behavior into extinction. The therapist, being a White male, also already carries considerable power and privilege in general within this context, and here he uses that to advocate the needs and treatment of his client who is not present. This therapist may then choose to further process what happened with his supervisor in individual supervision to navigate the other professional issues that arise from such public conflict with someone senior on the team, with whom the therapist shares a different power differential despite his own racial and gender privilege.

## COMMON CHALLENGES

The challenges inherent to this guideline around addressing and not perpetuating discrimination with our clients largely fall within our own emotional experience and reactions as therapists (see Box 6.2). This is why the self-reflection on and mindfulness of what we are experiencing internally as therapists are emphasized in this book. For instance, any of us who have committed a microaggression toward another (which I would predict is 100% of us) has likely experienced one of several key internal emotional reactions. First, a typical reaction that we have each likely experienced is defensiveness for whether we "meant" the received insult, typically with a justification of why we simply "could not have been racist/sexist/ageist/ableist, etc., because [insert all the ways we have shown our progressiveness with diversity issues professionally or personally]." This defensiveness is very natural and expected anytime we have been accused of any kind of character fault; however, in the clinical context, our defensiveness impedes our own ability to hold the dialectic between having done many actions that are in line with inclusion and equity to others *and yet* having just done something counter to that which actually caused harm or pain to our client, which in turn can impair our ability to address our own discriminatory actions as a therapist. Perhaps a helpful adage to keep in mind here is that it doesn't matter what you meant by what you said/ did, it matters how it felt to the person receiving it.

Second, for others (or perhaps following the initial bump of defensiveness) there are feelings of deep shame, guilt, or disappointment in ourselves for having done something discriminatory toward our client, and the discomfort we may feel with this realization in terms of its discrepancy to our core professional and personal values. These emotions are both valid and understandable, and likely will

---

Box 6.2

### COMMON CHALLENGES IN IMPLEMENTING GUIDELINE 6

* Feeling defensive about our intention when a client experiences a microaggression (committed by us as therapists)
* Such high feelings of shame or disappointment when we realize we have discriminated against a client, which is counter to our personal and professional values, to a level that prevents us from making amends
* Even upon making amends (as outlined in Exercise 6.1), the rupture is too great to overcome and the therapeutic alliance is irreversibly broken.
* Preemptively being so concerned about committing a microaggression with a client that it impairs your clinical services delivery
* Having a tendency to rationalize or explain a microaggression experience by our client by others ("cognitive restructuring mode").

---

help to propel us to make amends, but occasionally, individuals feel so ashamed that it impedes our ability to raise the misstep or address it with a client. This is problematic. I encourage you to review the skills and tips given in this chapter and accompanying resources to work on this strong emotional reaction and to consider that while it is difficult to feel such shame, **your client is the one who has been wronged**; as I said above, we have to dig deep into our resilience stores and address the issue to care for the person who came to us to provide a safe and therapeutic space, and we have an ethical responsibility as therapists to do so. That doesn't mean you don't also need your own support and work to deal with these strong feelings; but that needs to happen concurrently in your own support network (either personally or with professional assistance) while addressing the rupture with your client.

Now, being willing to be so vulnerable to address an act of discrimination perpetuated by you as the therapist also means an acceptance of the fact that even if you follow the steps provided in this chapter on working to repair the resulting rupture in alliance, your best efforts might work. Indeed, we can follow all the procedures for owning up to and trying to make amends for a committed microaggression, and the client can still not feel comfortable to continue with you or to be as open with you as is most therapeutically helpful. In this case, you have to work hard to ensure that they can see a therapist with whom they feel more comfortable, and share as little or as much as the client directs you to with that new provider, and ensure the client doesn't feel abandoned by you if you initiate this transfer, by explicitly sharing your fault in the clinical relationship as the reason for this referral and that the client was not in the wrong. **We have to take responsibility as the therapist for the rupture and make sure that the referral is not seen as punitive.** And then afterward, we should process this consequence of losing a client with our supervisors and peers, and learn from it for future clients. When such events occur, many of us do learn from it, but sometimes, we may also feel uncertain with future clients and may be inhibited in our clinical services out of fear of committing another microaggression. Similar to feelings of defensiveness or shame, this is a normal and understandable reaction; however, again, if this concern about committing a misstep impairs our clinical services delivery, we need to address that actively (either with our supervisors/peers, or in our own personal work with a therapist of our own).

Finally, sometimes it is difficult for us as therapists to switch out of our "protocol treatment" mode, and this can do a disservice to our clients. For instance, if a client reports having experienced an act of discrimination/microaggression by someone else outside of therapy, it is tempting to click into what I call "cognitive restructuring mode" where we want to automatically help the client reappraise the threat from that person perpetuating the discrimination and help them come up with possible alternative explanations or meanings for that person's actions. This can be very invalidating (as I have learned the hard way!), and Table 6.1 reminds us of how to navigate reports of discrimination in the most helpful and supportive way.

## PUTTING IT INTO PRACTICE

We have explored many skills together around this topic of microaggression and discrimination already in this book—and with good reason, because we do not typically receive much training in this domain, and if you're like me, you often feel the tension of recognizing the importance of the topic and yet not knowing what to do about it. Therefore, our practice section in this chapter (summarized in Box 6.3) is a review of what we have learned in this text so far. First, Table 6.1 can guide us in the process of assessing for the impact of discrimination and microaggressions on our clients, and building the rapport for clients to feel comfortable in continuing to bring up these issues in our work together.

Following this, Box 6.1 reminds us of the steps we can take to proactively prevent committing microaggressions toward our clients. Importantly, this process should be considered for *all* of our clients, not just those who are from minoritized backgrounds or simply different identity markers from our own; even if we identity as minorities ourselves, we are not immune to perpetuating microaggressions or discrimination toward others. Third, even if our best efforts are futile and we end up committing microaggressions toward our clients, we must recognize

---

Box 6.3

### How Do I Practice Guideline 6?

1. Use **Table 6.1** to guide your initial exploration with your client about their lived experiences of discrimination and/or microaggressions.
2. Review **Box 6.1** prior to starting with all clients (regardless of whether they match or differ on their intersectional identity factors from you) to mitigate the likelihood of committing a microaggression in therapy.
3. If a microaggression still occurs, walk through **Exercises 2.1 and 2.2** in full, and bring your reflections of these exercises to trusted peers or supervisors to consolidate what came up for you and to brainstorm most appropriate ways to proceed.
4. If you observe others committing a microaggression, use **Exercise 6.1** to help you become a more vocal advocate for the client being mistreated (whether they are physically present or not).
5. **Be brave** with your client if you are the perpetrator of discriminatory behavior: explicitly own your mistake, own the hurt it likely caused your client, and don't qualify/justify what you did. Practice in the mirror, in role-plays with colleagues, and then—do it. You can! You will probably feel poorly about yourself (shame, guilt, anger), and that is okay. If we act productively on such emotions by directly addressing our misstep, we can experience an important increase in our cultural humility and cultural competency.

---

the inevitable therapeutic rupture this will create. Exercises 2.1 and 2.2 from Chapter 2 on cultural humility (which can also be found in the Appendix) remind us how to repair such ruptures, which we are encouraged to bring back to trusted peers or supervisors who can provide us with our own safe space to navigate our reflections and reactions to committing such microaggressions. Exercise 6.1 in the current chapter guides us on ways to consider microaggressions we observe that are committed by others, which can be applied to both clinical team settings or within the context of group therapy.

Finally, we need to address the microaggression that has occurred (particularly when we are the offending party). This is probably the hardest piece for us as therapists: How do we admit that we, as individuals whose very role in the client's life is to provide safety, comfort, and support, have done something that could hurt our clients in such a fundamental way? I can only say the only way past something so painful for us as therapists is to go through it—bravely, fully owning the impact of our actions, and accepting the repercussions of what we did (including an acceptance of the fact that even with your best efforts, the rupture may not be fixable, but that is not a reason to not even try). We ask our clients to be vulnerable every time they step into our therapy room, and it feels uncomfortable for many therapists to also feel vulnerable in the therapy relationship, but we must remember that our discomfort (and shame, guilt, anger, whatever else we feel about our own actions, whether they were intentional or unintentional) pales in comparison to what the client likely felt as the recipient of such mistreatment. Through this process of explicitly owning and discussing what we did to repair and strengthen the alliance, we grow in our own cultural humility and cultural competency, and in keeping with the main theme of this book, we act as socially just mental health professionals in the process.

## COMMENTARY ON INCORPORATING SOCIAL JUSTICE

Indeed, the centrality of social justice approaches is imbued in every aspect of this guideline, as evident by my repeated reference to the importance of adopting this guideline in order to operate as socially just and equity-oriented therapists. That is, as we *recognize* and *label* observed microaggressions (whether perpetuated by ourselves or those we work with), we are in the position to better *address* such actions to ensure that harm to our clients, colleagues, and ourselves are minimized from the immediate insult, and to hopefully reduce the likelihood of a repeat offense. The other aspect of such efforts that I would like to further underscore here is that this effort is **everyone's responsibility**—not just those recognized as being dedicated to issues of equity and inclusion, not just to those who are visible or known minorities, not just to supervisors, not just to trainees, etc., but to every single one of us who have committed to bettering mental health for society by choosing to be psychologists. This is part of the very core of our ethical practice as mental health professionals, and if each of us stepped up to this often uncomfortable but crucial advocacy in whatever role we serve in this profession, our scientific field will be stronger and better for it, as will society and those we serve.

## DISCUSSION QUESTIONS

1. What are some examples you can recall where you were the recipient of discriminatory or microaggressive behavior? What did that bring up for you in terms of thoughts and feelings you were aware of in the moment, and later?

2. What are examples of when you perpetuated a microaggression, stereotyped someone, or witnessed it happening to someone else without speaking up? How did you feel in the moment and later? Were there any consequences?

3. What have you noticed about your own reactions to trainings and educational materials (even the content of this chapter) in the area of discrimination and how it pertains to clinical therapy? What personal life experiences or value systems do you think those reactions are stemming from? How does this impact the perspective you take as a therapist?

4. What do you struggle with in raising observed or committed microaggressions in supervisory, team, or training settings? How do others react, and what about that makes it harder or easier to address such issues in your practice setting?

5. **Social Justice Action**: What is one thing you can do in your current role (whatever stage of training or practice you are presently in) to commit to being an ally in your current practice setting to ensure that microaggressions do not occur in clinical team meetings or therapy sessions where you are present **this month**? How about at regular intervals moving forward? This can include working through exercises in this book, engaging in one or more of the listed resources around this topic, bringing in an invited speaker/trainer to your clinical setting on this topic, among many other options.

# 7

# Guideline 7

*Identifying and Incorporating Cultural Strengths
and Resources into Treatment*

## GUIDELINE 7 EXPLAINED

This guideline helpfully reminds us that a lot of what we consider to be "good" multicultural clinical practice is very much an extension of what is considered to be good overall clinical practice in our profession as therapists. In contemporary therapy approaches, we often talk about ensuring the incorporation of a patient's unique strengths into our treatments to maximize their effectiveness and client buy-in to the evidence-based strategies we teach. Within the context of culturally responsive treatment, the salient cultural or other identity factors themselves can be integrated as a core part of treatment if they are a major resource or impetus for positive change, and if belonging to a certain group provides an already existing extensive support network for the client (Cross, 2003).

Importantly, as we increase our engagement with communities more directly in our research and social justice work, we are more frequently reminded how culture itself can influence a range of culture-specific skills (e.g., Indigenous medicinal knowledge, cooking techniques and styles, agricultural practices), coping mechanisms (e.g., culture-specific metaphors for understanding psychological symptoms), interpersonal organizations and community resources (e.g., disability advocacy, religious or political activism, charitable community-focused events, cultural social events), and artistic outlets for emotion (through cultural expressions of dance, art, and music), all of which are prime avenues for exploration as a part of evidence-based practice (EBP) (Asnaani et al., 2022; Kaur et al., 2022).

For instance, within the context of a specific empirically supported treatment (EST) such as behavioral activation, culturally specific activities can be explicitly discussed and added to one's weekly activity of scheduling homework assignments. Similarly, for clients receiving exposure therapy for fear-based

*A Cultural Humility and Social Justice Approach to Psychotherapy.* Anu Asnaani, Oxford University Press.
© Oxford University Press 2023. DOI: 10.1093/oso/9780197635971.003.0008

disorders, hierarchy items that directly link to cultural activities that have been avoided by the client due to the anxiety symptoms they elicit can be added to increase both buy-in to exposure practice and the immediate benefit of engaging in such activities, extending beyond just habituation to fear. More broadly, aligning specific activities with one's core cultural values (for those identifying such values as inherently meaningful) can be utilized in any of the values-focused treatment approaches, such as mindfulness and values exploration or acceptance and commitment therapy. Indeed, incorporating a client's culture-based skill sets and activities into EBP can be a way to improve adherence to between-session treatment homework to provide a desirable context in which to practice therapy skills, and to bolster the client's intrinsic motivation for doing so.

That said, inquiring about a client's culturally influenced strengths and resources may not be as straightforward as one might imagine, since there is variability in how acceptable direct inquiry to clients about their own strengths may be. For instance, Hays (2009) wisely advises that certain cultures in specific geographical regions or Indigenous backgrounds (e.g., those identifying as aligning most closely with certain Asian or Native American cultural values) are culturally socialized to show modesty around individual strengths, and therefore, a client may find it challenging to verbalize their own strengths if such individuals are directly questioned about this area. One suggested work-around for this issue, to obtain information that can be incorporated into treatment, is to ask the individual to think about what others in their social or family circles might say are the client's strengths or core culturally based motivations. This could be a particularly helpful way to gain insight on possible cultural resources for treatment integration if it is clear from your culturally informed assessment of the client that they have a more interdependent cultural orientation in which others' opinions are highly valued.

In general, finding ways to incorporate culture-influenced strengths, practices, activities, and support systems into the EBP approach can be highly therapeutic and reinforcing of adherence to prescribed treatment skills (e.g., integration of American Indian/Alaskan Native traditional practices into substance use treatment and motivational interviewing approaches for adolescents from this community; Dickerson, Brown, Johnson, Schweigman, & D'Amico, 2016). The balance that the therapist needs to strike here is ensuring that such integration of cultural strengths and resources does not integrally change the core mechanism of change that the chosen evidence-based treatment is intended to have, or avoids the crucial points of intervention, thereby undermining the intended effectiveness of the treatment (Asnaani & Hofmann, 2012).

Box 7.1 provides some ways to assess for such culturally relevant strengths and resources, and then our Case Application for this chapter provides an applied model for how we may utilize such prompts and subsequent information about the client's culturally relevant strengths while not threatening the core psychotherapy strategies used.

Box 7.1

PROMPTS TO ASSESS FOR CULTURALLY RELEVANT STRENGTHS AND RESOURCES

Consider the following questions that you may pose to clients to more explicitly raise the possibility of incorporating culturally relevant strengths across some different types of ESTs (note: this is a subsample, not an exhaustive list of ESTs, and you're encouraged to think about how these can be modified for other treatment approaches):

* **Broad prompts to explore**: *What would you say are your strengths, talents, or abilities that people in your family, community, or social network recognize, value, or appreciate about you? What do others in your life say you're good at? What do you believe you bring to relationships with others that you see as a positive part of who you are or what you're capable of? This can be in terms of certain skills you are known to be good at/you feel that you're good at, personality characteristics you are valued for in your family/community, or certain knowledge that you can contribute to certain situations that maybe others don't have as much of.* [THEN THIS INFORMATION CAN BE USED FOR ANY OF THE MORE EST-SPECIFIC PROMPTS BELOW.]

* **For behavioral activation approaches**: *As we think about ways to help increase your daily pleasure and motivation, it sometimes helps to include activities that are personally relevant for us so we feel more genuinely motivated to do them. For instance, I have had clients mention that certain cultural practices, political or social activism, religious involvement, or specific family activities, just to name a few examples, are some things that they used to feel a lot of joy about doing before they got depressed. Are there any activities that are maybe connected to specific parts of your life or identities that we should consider adding into your weekly activity scheduling?*

* **For exposure therapy approaches**: *It's sometimes helpful for us to put items on our exposure hierarchies that allow us to face our fears to do something that is personally relevant to us or tied to a bigger part of ourselves, like maybe a community we belong to, something particularly important to our families, or something that is connected to or affirms a part of our identity. Can you think of any things you're avoiding that are particularly upsetting because they are otherwise really important to you and that you would do if you didn't feel anxious?*

* **For cognitive therapy approaches**: *You have mentioned that your family/community is pretty aware that you often have depressive/suicidal/anxious thoughts. What are some ways that your loved ones have helped you gently challenge those thoughts in a way that doesn't feel judgmental but, instead, supportive? I often observe that there are some nuggets of wisdom in the ways our communities/families try to support us when we have difficult thoughts,*

*and I'd love to explore if we could use any of those helpful approaches as we practice cognitive restructuring/challenging in our work together.*

* **For mindfulness and values-based approaches**: *As we explore the values that are most personally relevant to us and that we want to live our lives by, it is undeniable that our identities, whether it's our particular cultural background, gender, religion, age, sexual orientation, or any number of identity factors that make us who we are, can influence what values are most important to us. While I want to encourage you to think about what values are most important to you (and not just your family/community), I completely get that for many of us, our values are greatly connected to those specific parts of our identities that are most important to us. I'd love for this to be a space where we can talk about what you have noticed about some of your own strengths in your family and community systems, and how these might be connected to how you want to be in the world and the values that are most important to you. What might some of those strengths that you value in your relationships within your community or shared community values be that you hold in high regard?* [IDEALLY EXPLICITLY NAME THE IDENTITY FACET(S) THAT THE CLIENT HAS ALREADY RAISED AS MOST SALIENT INSTEAD OF USING SUCH GENERAL TERMS HERE.]

* **For relapse prevention phases of treatment**: *In order to maintain all the progress you have made in therapy, it's helpful for us to keep thinking about how you can practice what you have learned here in areas that are personally relevant to you, even long after therapy is done.* [RETURN TO FIRST BROAD PROMPT, AND DISCUSS APPLICATION OF IDENTIFIED STRENGTHS/RESOURCES CONNECTED TO IDENTITY FACETS IN THE SHORT, MEDIUM, AND LONG TERM.]

---

## CASE APPLICATION

*Case description.* For the application of this guideline, let's return to Massie, our 46-year-old, divorced, nonbinary, bisexual, Filipinx-American, Catholic client (first introduced in Chapter 2). Massie presents with a number of diverse intersectional identity factors based on their cultural and religious backgrounds, single-parent status of two teenage children, and gender identity/sexual orientation, and all these present potential avenues to incorporate identity-related strengths into treatment of their primary symptoms of depression and generalized anxiety. As a reminder, Massie's family and faith/cultural communities are mixed in their reactions to their recently disclosed sexual orientation. For instance, their children have no issue with it, and their parents seem similarly supportive. However, their extended family members and certain members of their church are quite unsupportive about both their divorce and various queer identities, which complicates their utilization as positive resources to incorporate into their treatment, despite both family and faith being important elements identified by Massie in their life.

*Evidence-based treatment approach.* Given the primary symptoms of major depression and generalized anxiety disorder, the therapist took a phased approach to treatment for Massie. First, the basic principles of behavioral activation (a front-line treatment for depression; Martell, Dimidjian, & Herman-Dunn, 2010) were introduced early in treatment, to orient the client to the importance of actively scheduling activities that have been pleasurable in the past (whether or not they are currently associated with enjoyment or pleasure) in order to improve mood, with psychoeducation around the utility of such an approach presented in the first few sessions. The second phase, which involved more directed treatment for generalized anxiety, was gradually brought in after the first 4–6 sessions, and consisted of a values-based and mindfulness approach as the evidence-based treatment (Roemer & Orsillo, 2020). Briefly, this approach entails psychoeducation around the importance of building a present-centered awareness, and encourages reflection on one's core values to guide subsequent action and life goals. This treatment, from my perspective, nicely dovetails and complements behavioral activation in the case of co-morbid depression and chronic worry because it continues to encourage the client to be active in their daily lives, using one's own values as the inspiration for what that activity is chosen to be, rather than external expectations. Such an approach might be particularly beneficial for someone like Massie who receives conflicting messages about what parts of their life and identity are acceptable to those surrounding them.

*Preamble to therapy dialogue.* Within this session, the therapist's first task will be to work with Massie to figure out which parts of their identity are most salient to them, to identify potentially adaptive behavioral activation targets for their depression, and/or values-based action for addressing their chronic worry. It is essential that the client has the buy-in to incorporate these identity-based activities or facets into the treatment, and providing choice can further empower the client to engage in these therapeutic targets. Let's see how the therapist navigates this line of inquiry.

> **Therapist**: *Massie, it's been so great to see you start to rebuild activities in your life that used to be things you did before the depression started. How has it felt to start scheduling in things that used to bring you pleasure into your week?*
>
> **Massie**: *It's been fine. I still don't really enjoy doing any of them, though. I sort of just am going through the motions, but I guess I feel a bit better about the fact that I'm at least doing some things now that I haven't done for a while, like reading more or cooking with my kids. They like that at least.*
>
> **Therapist**: *I agree that it's great that you're doing more of what you have been wanting to, although I'm sorry it's still not bringing you the pleasure or lifting your mood in the way we had hoped. That's not very unusual; sometimes when we start re-engaging in previously pleasurable activities, our bodies and moods take a bit of time to catch up. I have been wondering if maybe one way we can help it along and make these efforts even more valuable to you is to think about activities we*

*can schedule that are related to other parts of your life that are important to you. For instance, you have brought up here that coming out, while it has been difficult, has also been really freeing for you, and I'm curious, have there been any activities around queer activism or queer pride that you have been wanting to engage in or used to enjoy being active in before the depression and worries took hold?*

**Massie**: *Mmm, not really. I am proud to be out, but don't feel a big need right now to be very outspoken or anything about it.*

**Therapist**: *Okay, that makes sense. I'm just throwing out some ideas here, and you can completely say those aren't of interest, but if something I mention sounds like a potential way for us to incorporate some more meaningful activities into our weekly homework, just say the word, okay? Sometimes my clients mention enjoying cultural activities, like celebrating certain festivals, being involved in community events, things like that. Or, getting involved in their faith community in some way. Or even just being more social with other like-minded people, like maybe a single parents' group or trying to get into another social circle for both support and company. Do any of these sound like something you want more of in your life, or something else entirely?*

**Massie**: *Well, of all of those, I do have an interest in becoming more active at church again, because that part of my life took a big hit when I came out. And maybe getting more involved in some more Filipino activities, for the sake of my kids.*

**Therapist**: *Wonderful—I'd love to hear a bit more about those so we can see if there's something there we can add to your weekly activities list. Let's start with the church part—I know you have mentioned that there were members of your church who were less than kind about you coming out, but I think you mentioned there were some folks who were supportive, weren't there? In what capacity do you remember being supported when at church, or in what type of specific church contexts or settings?*

**Massie**: *It was definitely when I was part of the choir, basically my whole choir was behind me, and once I started singing, all the awkwardness of knowing everyone knew I was queer just melted away [sighs]. I miss that. With the divorce and coming out and everything, I just sort of stopped going.*

**Therapist**: *Hmm, that must have been so hard to lose something you love like singing in the choir on top of everything else. I wonder, what do you think about potentially approaching the choir leader to see if you can perhaps rejoin? I just think that if we incorporate an activity that used to bring you significant joy before the depression started, that you might experience a greater improvement in your mood than you're currently getting from our activity scheduling. What do you think?*

**Massie**: *It's hard to imagine ever being that happy again as I was when we would all sing, but I know that would make me feel great if it did. I'm definitely willing to at least ask if there is any spot still open and if they'll have me back. I think they would, they were sad to see me go.*

**Therapist**: *Great—I think it's worth a shot, right? So, why don't we set that as one thing you'll do this week, to at least reach out to the choir leader to explore that possibility. I think that's a great plan. Now, for the Filipino activities bit, let's explore the options there. Just so I understand what parts of the cultural practices are most important to you, what makes you most excited or happy about your cultural background that you want your kids to experience, too?*

**Massie**: *I mean, there are a bunch of things, but food for sure! [laughs]. I'm already cooking with my kids, but I don't tend to do Filipino food, even though I know we'd all enjoy it. But my kids say I'm a good cook, so I think with some recipes or guidance I might be able to figure it out and then they'll remember their heritage that way.*

**Therapist**: *Food is a great place to start, and it sounds like you have the advantage of being a good cook on your side! And what I like about this activity is that it also aligns with some of the other values-based work we have started doing more recently, because I remember you stating that you wanted to be a good parent, one that your children can rely on and look up to, and I wonder if passing on parts of your Filipino heritage in this way is in line with being a good parent, you know what I mean? Let's chat about ways we can already incorporate that value-based activity in the coming week, whether through getting some recipes or having your mom call in to guide you all through some tasty recipes of foods you used to particularly enjoy or think the kids might enjoy learning to make with you. What do you think is the best way to try to tap into that part of your cultural background this week?*

*Summary of guideline application.* As seen in the way this exchange progresses, the therapist offers some examples of identity-based activities that may still fit with the evidence-based strategy (behavioral activation and/or values-based action), but then gives the client full domain over what resonates the most with them. Further, she highlights what the client's overall strengths are, to further motivate them to take these steps (e.g., reflecting back how much the client enjoyed singing in the choir and what a good cook they are). Incorporating activities that are integrally linked to the identity facets that the client currently most values into specific homework targets may allow the client to really be more motivated overall and to derive greater secondary benefits to engaging in behavioral activation or values-based action, thereby targeting their depression and chronic worry symptoms even more effectively.

## COMMON CHALLENGES

One of the biggest challenges to incorporating cultural strengths into EBPs is not being sure how to do so in a way that does not influence the actual active ingredients or strategies of your intervention (see Box 7.2). This is particularly challenging for many clinicians because the majority of our protocol treatments do not give clear guidelines for how to integrate cultural factors into treatment

Box 7.2

## Common Challenges in Implementing Guideline 7

* Lack of clarity around how to assess and then actually incorporate cultural strengths and resources in a way that does not threaten the active ingredients of your EBP
* Concern about overemphasizing culturally relevant activities in your intervention, coming across as stereotyping of your client based on their identity facets
* Client being reticent to share their own strengths as they pertain to identity factors, or finding it hard to verbalize/identify such strengths, even from a loved one's perspective as recommended
* Disagreement with client about what culturally related activities are likely to be therapeutic in the context of therapy and which ones may be partially contributing to presenting symptoms or may impede with therapy skills practice.

---

strategies (hence the need for this book!). That said, most protocols do, in fact, at least prescribe what the theoretical and empirical mechanisms for each treatment are, and this is where we could benefit from taking the individual-specific cultural factors raised by our clients and interlaying them upon the active treatment strategies prescribed by specific ESTs. One way to assist us in doing such culturally responsive EBP is to consult with colleagues and supervisors about what general treatment categories each of our identified cultural strengths may fall into (e.g., can we use the strength as a means for behavioral activation, or is it better suited as being an item on an exposure hierarchy?), as we discuss in the next section on practicing this skill and as exemplified by the Case Application for this chapter.

The second area of hesitation often observed in clinicians attempting to integrate culture-specific resources and strengths into treatment is a concern around doing so in a culturally insensitive way or appearing as stereotyping of a client based on their explicit identity factors. This is a challenge that can be directly addressed by the skill we discuss in Chapter 2 on cultural humility—practicing being vulnerable around our own lack of knowledge and taking a curious, respectful approach with our clients. Specifically, being explicit with this concern with clients (see suggested prompts and explanations for this effort in Box 7.1), working with your client to ensure that there is buy-in from your client to incorporate such cultural strengths or resources into treatment (and backing off from doing so if there is not).

Then we run into the challenge that clients (while they may show under-standing for how incorporating such culturally specific activities could be helpful for their treatment) may be either reticent to share personally relevant examples of such activities, or they even find it difficult to verbalize/identify such strengths and recognize such attributes in themselves. I recommend that one way to get around this barrier is to enlist the perspective of a loved one who may be better positioned to recognize and identify such strengths (e.g., *"I remember when XXX used to love doing YYY, but since they have been feeling anxious/depressed/using substances, they have not been engaging in this activity, which is a shame because they used to be really great at it."*). However, some-times loved ones may be either inaccessible or themselves unable to identify such cultural strengths. In this case, there may need to be more time allowed to have the client reflect on their identities more broadly (What are the positively regarded elements related to their diverse identity facets that they want more of in their life? What have been times in the past, even the distant past, where they found joy or strength from a cultural activity/engagement?). Then the therapist can leverage such a broader exploration/reflection into identifying specific ways to incorporate culturally specific experiences and activities into the treatment.

Finally, it is not unlikely that we will occasionally differ from our clients around what culturally specific activities or resources they regard as positive and which we instead regard as potentially problematic in terms of maintaining or exacerbating their presenting problem. For instance, a client may identify en-gagement in a particular community group as a source of social support, while that same group may have members who are disparaging against the client getting mental health treatment or who are exacerbating the client's symptoms because of their repeated negative interpersonal interactions with the client. In this case, we need to proceed cautiously. On the one hand, we do not want to of-fend the client or remove some foundational pillars of their connection to their community, and yet we do not want to push for increased engagement in an activity that may threaten their progress in treatment. If such a situation occurs, the client can be engaged in an open conversation about what parts of that par-ticular cultural activity/resource are seen as positive and supportive of emotional health, and what parts they regard as potentially problematic (with some gentle suggestions from the therapist if none is identified by the client). The therapist can acknowledge the importance of this identified cultural activity or resource and still strategically focus on incorporating other ones deemed to be more in line with therapeutic recovery, ideally in agreement with the client so that this process is as transparent as possible and the client is empowered as an equal agent in this process.

Box 7.3

## How Do I Practice Guideline 7?

1. First **assess** for potential cultural sources and examples of resources, strengths, and activities related to salient identity characteristics which may be good candidates to incorporate into treatment (see Exercise 7.1 for sample assessment prompts).
2. **Categorize** what part of your treatment protocol or process the identified cultural strength or resource may best fit (as part of core intervention or as reward for treatment engagement?). Consult with peers, supervisors, and experts to figure this out.
3. **Openly discuss with your client** how you think these activities may be integrated into your treatment based on what you come up with in step 2. Get your client's input on how to most effectively and acceptably do this.
4. **Periodically assess** the utility of incorporating such culturally relevant resources into your treatment, and how it may be even qualitatively related to a range of outcomes for the client. Use Exercise 7.1 as a guide when needed through various stages of treatment.

## PUTTING IT INTO PRACTICE

When we think about practice of this specific guideline, there are two levels (see Box 7.3). First, how do we go about assessing for culturally relevant strengths and resources that may be relevant to incorporate into our treatment, both practically and in a culturally responsive, non-stereotyping way? To this end, Box 7.1 and the Case Application provide some ways to do so, addressing both the specific questions we can ask and how to phrase such questions and the rationale provided to clients about why we are exploring this area (i.e., to augment and enhance the treatment) and how it relates to their target symptoms (i.e., better symptom reduction or increased quality of life).

The second level that naturally follows assessment is ensuring that we can then effectively utilize this information to enhance our EBP, and this can lead us to wonder, how do we make it an integral part of our treatment approach? This part of the skill requires a bit more creativity, consultation, and reflection, both on the part of the therapist (primarily) and also on the client (occasionally). The first step of this process is to categorize the identified cultural strengths, resources, or activities: Are they potential avenues in which to deliver core strategies of your chosen EST (e.g., potential exposure hierarchy items), or are they positive reinforcers/rewards (i.e., will they bring intrinsic joy/pleasure or desired social engagement to the client without generating much negative affect) for behavior change/engagement in your prescribed therapeutic strategies? To figure this out, you may have to consult with a supervisor or peer, or a colleague who either has more expertise in culturally responsive treatments or expertise in the particular EST you are employing.

Then, depending on which broad area of treatment you think this identified strength may be better suited to (intervention avenue versus being a positive consequence), it is important to have an explicit and collaborative conversation with your client regarding your suggestions about how to incorporate this information into one of those two domains. This allows you as the therapist to elicit their feedback on how this can be practically done, as they are the experts on their own cultural identity backgrounds and communities, and to ensure that no other avenues were left unexplored as a better match for such treatment incorporation. Once this has been discussed and there is consensus, you and the client can implement the chosen activity, resource, or strength in the agreed-upon domain.

Finally, the scientist in me would encourage you as the therapist to periodically assess how useful it was to incorporate such culturally relevant facets into treatment for the client in terms of addressing their symptoms, quality of life, and overall cultural identification. This can be in the form of unstructured debriefing as treatment progresses (ideally, so that other areas for expansion or modification of this effort to support treatment progress can be assessed), or at the end of treatment to help both the therapist and client understand how treatment was most helpful and how this learning can be consolidated or strengthened even after treatment concludes (see brief mention of this in Box 7.1 and more on this in Chapter 8 on incorporating our guidelines into relapse prevention to maintain treatment gains). In addition, Exercise 7.1 presents a handy checklist that outlines these various steps discussed in this section as a quick self-assessment during practice of this skill.

Exercise 7.1

CHECKLIST WORKSHEET FOR INCORPORATING IDENTIFIED IDENTITY-
RELATED STRENGTHS AND RESOURCES INTO TREATMENT

Did I (check each one as you complete, ideally chronologically):

☐ **Assess for identity-related strengths/resources that may be incorporated into treatment?**

Which ones, specifically?

☐ Culture-specific skills and knowledge (e.g., community naturalistic/
medicinal health expertise, cooking, storytelling)

☐ Culture-specific coping strategies (e.g., cultural metaphors for understanding emotional symptoms, interpersonal activities that are culturally relevant or valued)

☐ Specific community resources (e.g., identity-related political or social
causes, places for worship, or financial resources)

☐ Artistic outlets for processing of emotional material (e.g., culture-
specific dance, art, and music)

☐ **Work with peers/supervisors and do my own assessment of which specific parts of my current EST protocol would be most appropriate to
incorporate identified strengths?**

☐ **Broach the topic and explain the rationale to the client so they are
empowered and informed about my intention to bring such identity-
related strengths into our work together?**

**Have I continued to check in with client about using such specific identity-
related strengths, resources, or activities after our initial conversation?**

☐ Yes, I have brought up the topic again after the first time.

☐ No, I have not revisited the topic.

If not, why haven't I done so? _____

_____

Do I need to reconsider bringing it up again? When might it be helpful to consider
doing so?

_____

_____

_____

## COMMENTARY ON INCORPORATING SOCIAL JUSTICE

When we engage our clients in generating unique and personally relevant ways to practice the evidence-based strategies we teach (whether these constitute values-based action, behavioral activation, or something else), we are in essence engaging them as equal partners in their own recovery, which is a core tenet of many of our contemporary psychology approaches. Indeed, making the distinct effort to veer away from our prepared list of prescribed activities that have been typically informed by treatment of clients with specific demographics (i.e., White, middle-class, cis-gendered, and heterosexual clients), we are showing in our practice that we value the diverse identities of our clients and empower them to bring these identities into our treatment and implementation of evidence-based skills. I have been struck at the number of times I have handed out standard activity checklists from behavioral activation protocols in various community settings only to have my client blankly stare back at me because none of the suggested activities is congruent with what brings them joy or meaning in their own lives. That said, such checklists have been utilized to help jump-start a client's own thinking about activities they wish to engage in, and so using our own cultural knowledge and some of the worksheets in this chapter can help us generate a list that might be more likely to "land" with clients of diverse backgrounds. In this way, we can rely on the utility of why such lists were generated to begin with, in order to help our clients get the most out of such skills, and to ensure that we incorporate their own cultural strengths and preferences most effectively into treatment.

## DISCUSSION QUESTIONS

1. What are some resources, activities, or strengths that you are aware of or that are pertinent to your own cultural or identity background that you have relied on to support your own or your loved ones' mental health? How could you envision such facets being integrated into the types of evidence-based treatments you have most typically employed with clients?
2. What is an example of a time when your client either independently incorporated such culturally related resources or activities into your work together, or that you realize now in retrospect could have been more centrally integrated into your work with a particular client?
3. What do you feel unsure or uncertain about in terms of incorporating such elements into either core parts of your treatment or as an explicit reward/facilitator of your work with a client? How can you address these internal barriers to practicing this skill?
4. How would your supervisors and peers in your current practice setting respond to such an approach as prescribed in the current guideline? If you are concerned that there may be some pushback on doing so, what

is most likely to be the reason for resistance to this approach in your current setting? (Is it about taking too much time in session to explore such potential resources with clients, or concerns about how it may negatively impact the core evidence-based strategy you are supposed to employ, or something else?)

5. **Social Justice Action**: Considering any resistance in your current practice setting (or training program), what can you do to advocate for your clients and to explain why encouraging and supporting clients in using culturally relevant activities and resources would serve as a worthwhile integration into your clinical approach with your trainers/trainees, clinic administrators, and colleagues?

# 8

# Utilizing the Guidelines to Enhance Relapse Prevention and Maintenance of Treatment Gains

Now that all seven guidelines have been explained and exemplified, we turn to a few last issues to consider within the therapy course, with a focus in this chapter on how we can (and should) utilize the guidelines within the context of relapse prevention as treatment draws to the end and in helping clients maintain their gains in therapy after therapy has concluded. Indeed, this final phase of treatment is central to preventing recurrence or re-emergence of a range of psychological symptoms in a number of treatment protocols (Witkiewitz & Marlatt, 2007), and with good reason. Relapse-prevention efforts in the context of evidence-based therapy is crucial because it provides a safety net of sorts to our clients, providing guidance on how they may utilize what they have learned in therapy as they end their time with us in therapy, to anticipate the challenges or life events that may re-trigger their symptoms to a problematic level, and to fully realize how they can be their own therapists to manage any re-emergence or worsening of symptoms as they progress through their lives.

Indeed, despite our best efforts as mental health practitioners, relapse rates for many common psychological symptoms are significant (although variable; for instance, around 30% for depression in adults, but only 8%–10% for children and young adults with anxiety disorders; Levy, Stevens, & Tolin, 2021). In addition, recurrence of mental health symptoms is associated with considerable burden both to the individual (e.g., higher yearly personal healthcare costs) and to the society/healthcare system at large (e.g., higher healthcare resource utilization such as greater emergency room visits and inpatient admissions) (Gauthier, Mucha, Shi, & Guerin, 2019).

*A Cultural Humility and Social Justice Approach to Psychotherapy.* Anu Asnaani, Oxford University Press.
© Oxford University Press 2023. DOI: 10.1093/oso/9780197635971.003.0009

Thus, it's clear that relapse prevention is important, but how do our culturally competent treatment practices and guidelines that we have discussed in detail fit into this final phase of treatment? My answer is: they fit integrally into the whole process of relapse prevention. Indeed, data indicate that individuals from diverse identity backgrounds (i.e., those identifying as ethnic/racial minorities, lower socioeconomic status, sexual/gender minorities, etc.) are more likely to show first episodes and/or recurrence of symptoms of various internalizing and externalizing disorders after treatment (e.g., Levy et al., 2021; Burcasa & Iacono, 2007). To be clear, these higher rates and severity of symptoms are likely not driven by simply being of a diverse identity background. Rather, this observation is likely directly driven by external sociopolitical determinants that maintain significant health disparities in many of these groups (e.g., a greater exposure to stressful life events, less equitable access to good evidence-based treatments; Derr, 2016; Gutierrez Chavez et al., 2022), which I would hypothesize could potentially impact relapse and one's maintenance of gains from treatment. The guidelines we discuss in this book allow us to strengthen our individual relationships with our diverse clients, which we hope, in turn, would positively impact the likelihood that clients will continue to use the skills they learned in therapy effectively. In addition, the guidelines remind us how we may alter the broader therapeutic climate that perpetuates inequitable care for diverse groups to reduce relapse on a larger scale, by charging us with social justice action items we can pursue to address such disparities in clinical care.

Further, while I have referred to relapse prevention in the individual guideline chapters occasionally, I want to provide a bit more consolidated narrative here about how we can concretely use our guidelines to enhance and broaden the scope of relapse prevention. I discuss this next, followed by a brief Case Application to show these guidelines in action specifically within the context of relapse prevention. I also provide a worksheet that allows us to plan which guidelines will be most relevant (and how) before our relapse-prevention sessions as we near the end of therapy with a particular client.

## INCORPORATING OUR GUIDELINES INTO RELAPSE PREVENTION

From our seven guidelines, several stand out as particularly relevant to the discussion of relapse prevention. First, Guideline 2 ("Practicing Cultural Humility as a Continuous Process") certainly applies to this final phase of treatment. As we work with the client to explore what parts of their lives would require continuous application of therapy skills even as treatment ends, we need to be open and honest about our own gaps in knowledge about how some of the work can be applied across cultural situations that might arise for the client. For instance, did we discuss certain activities within the context of behavioral activation for depression that just might not be feasible or acceptable when our client is at home in their more rural setting? This process of being mindful, being open to getting it wrong, and eliciting the client's equal participation in thinking how the skills will most readily apply to their lives when therapy is finished continues to be a high priority in this phase, to ensure the client knows how to continue using their skills in the most effective and feasible way.

This guideline dovetails nicely in this way with Guideline 4 ("Engaging in Self-Education about Specific Cultural Norms Using a Variety of Sources"), so that we don't necessarily put the entire burden of trying to figure out how these therapy skills will be fully and independently incorporated by our clients in their cultural/identity contexts on our clients themselves. This would be another great opportunity to pull in a community leader, trusted family member, or a cultural expert/consultant, and to work with them to better appreciate the ways to ensure that the treatment strategies can stand on their own without regular guidance from a therapist in these various contexts. For instance, what is expected might change in your client's role as they progress in age or family expansion by their religious faith (e.g., are there specific religious rites/ceremonies that might come up later that could trigger their social anxiety significantly, or expectations for how they raise their children within a particular faith, or choose a partner, even if they are not at those stages yet?). Helping your client consider how specific and expected cultural events may ignite their symptoms will empower them to be ready to address them head-on as they occur, hopefully reducing the likelihood of considerable dysfunction as a result. We are likely not going to be aware of such future events, and considering a range of sources to educate ourselves on these will allow us to guide our clients more effectively on what to expect and how to manage their symptoms when these occur.

Of course, along with discussing specific cultural milestones or events that might require particular use of therapy skills, such a conversation should include a discussion about what other cultural barriers (as we explored in Guideline 5) may interfere with use of therapeutic skills, and what impact future instances of discrimination/microaggressions (as we explored in Guideline 6) may have on the client's symptoms and ability to employ their therapy skills to manage their mental health. For instance, as our adolescent client returns to their friend group in high school or college and they mention having been in therapy or using a skill they learned previously in therapy when treatment is already complete, what do they do if they are faced with derogatory or stigmatizing words about having been in therapy? What if they are personally verbally insulted, or it is insinuated, directly or indirectly, that they are weak or "losers" for having received therapy? By proactively thinking through how such barriers can impact their willingness to use adaptive skills to manage their symptoms, and how they can protect themselves from having such acts of discrimination take away their self-efficacy in using their therapy skills, we allow clients to be more ready to address the various types of events that can detract from the long-term effectiveness of a treatment they have benefited from in the acute treatment phase.

Finally, we can use Guideline 7 to figure out the specific identity-based strengths and resources that a client can use to expand and consolidate their learning in therapy, a skill we do discuss a bit more directly within the context of relapse prevention in that chapter. For instance, is there an area that aligns with both their core values (such as advocacy or social fairness) and a particular aspect of their identity (such as having a disability) so that we can come up with a plan for them to pursue in a phased and growing fashion, even long after therapy is completed? Working with our clients to think about broader activities that integrate personally relevant activities and allow them to continue to apply their therapy skills (such as a commitment to core values, as is often used in acceptance-based approaches for anxiety) can be really powerful in ensuring they stay connected to continuous and meaningful application of the tools they picked up in therapy.

Let's look at some of these in action in our Case Application that explores relapse-prevention planning with our case Tess, to briefly provide an exemplar of how we can raise some of these guidelines within this final phase of treatment. Following this, Exercise 8.1 provides a checklist of the guidelines with spaces for you to fill in the blanks of specific ways to incorporate each guideline during relapse prevention planning for your own individual client.

## CASE APPLICATION

*Case description.* As you may recall from Chapter 3, Tess is our 24-year-old, Latina, straight, cis-gendered woman who immigrated from El Salvador as a teenager who is currently pursuing a graduate degree in accounting. She presents to treatment with symptoms of panic disorder with agoraphobia, specifically reporting sudden bouts of intense crying, acute anxiety, heat in the chest that radiates to her head, and significant avoidance of public places that she has deemed the most "risky" where such "emotion attacks" (as she calls them) are most likely to occur (e.g., supermarket, department stores, and bridges). As we discussed previously, she lives near her uncle and his family in a major U.S. city, but she has several younger brothers and her father still living in El Salvador, all of whom she has not been able to see due to complications with her DACA immigration status. She has a good social circle consisting of both Latine and non-Latine friends, but often feels disconnected from her mother, who doesn't speak English or understand Tess's educational aspirations or delay in starting to have paid work, which causes significant interpersonal tension and feelings of guilt for Tess.

*Evidence-based treatment approach.* The chosen treatment approach closely resembles a front-line CBT protocol for panic and agoraphobia (e.g., the protocol prescribed by Craske & Barlow, 2007). As we discussed in Chapter 3, this treatment includes first providing psychoeducation around the function of anxiety/panic, assisting in the identification of unhelpful thoughts that may maintain the anxiety and subsequent avoidance (e.g., "something is physically wrong with me" or "if I'm alone in a supermarket, this is unsafe because I might panic"), followed by encouragement of the client to gradually approach their feared situations via in vivo exposures, and interoceptive exposures, which entails repeated, purposeful induction of physical symptoms of anxiety. Treatment typically occurs once a week for the standard session of 45–60 minutes and concludes after 10–15 weekly sessions.

*Preamble to therapy dialogue.* At this stage of treatment, we have successfully treated Tess's presenting symptoms of panic disorder with agoraphobia with cognitive therapy and interoceptive/in vivo exposure as described above. Over the course of therapy, we have explored culturally laden themes related to her immigrant status, acculturative stress, strains on her family relationships, and her culturally congruent definitions of what she is experiencing in terms of her emotional health. As we enter this last stage of treatment, the therapist has gone through the checklist of guidelines, recognizing that several will be important to keep at the forefront when setting up the relapse-prevention plan with Tess. The guidelines the therapist is referring to with each part of the following dialogue (Guidelines 4–6) are indicated in the exchange. We join the conversation immediately following their review of what Tess found useful or helpful in therapy as the therapist pivots the session to future planning to keep up the use of her skills after therapy ends and prevent a problematic return of her symptoms.

**Therapist:** *Tess, you have done so well with treatment, and I'm so glad to hear that you have also found some of the things we learned in therapy to be helpful for you in reducing your current symptoms and for managing your stress more generally. As you get ready to end therapy, I want us to think about how we might want to take these lessons learned forward in your life and continue practicing your skills so we can keep your symptoms down, even as other stressful events come up. One of the things I would love to learn more about from you is about whether there are any family events or significant stages in your family's immigration story that might come up for you over the next few years as you complete graduate school? My reason for asking about this is to help us think ahead about what might be an added stress to the already stressful context of trying to finish your degree, so we can have a plan in place to manage it.*

[GUIDELINE 4: Engaging in self-education about specific cultural norms using a variety of sources]

**Tess:** *Oh, yes, I understand. Well, we're waiting every day to see when we might get a breakthrough in getting my father and brothers up here, and it all depends on getting this one document that will allow us to at least bring them here legally, since it's been such a hassle to get our papers done here for my mom and me. And of course, I'm still on DACA status, which is stressful at certain times when there is a change in government because I don't know if I'll lose my status. So, there are things that can lead to stress, but I can't quite anticipate when those come up.*

**Therapist**: *That makes a lot of sense, and I can get how both of those events can be stressful, and yet unpredictable. And one thing we learned about your panic is that you don't love that it's unpredictable to begin with, yes? Although, you have done amazingly in tolerating the uncertainty through your in vivo exposure, and I expect this will continue to be important if these events arise. For instance, we can write down the steps you should take if these events suddenly occur and you start to notice an increase in your panic or avoidance symptoms. In addition, remember how we talked about there being a greater likelihood that you will experience a panic attack if your overall stress level is higher? If that happens, we want to automatically (whether you notice the stress level increase right away or not) switch into some of those general stress-management techniques we discussed: eating regularly, getting enough sleep, connecting with your friends, getting enough exercise, and so on. Also, we might want to immediately get some advice or feedback from the immigration services agency you have been working with to get guidance on how to navigate your own DACA status, just to get some additional professional support. What else can you think of, and what are some ways to make sure you use your skills proactively when those immigration stressors come up?* [THERAPIST GUIDES CLIENT THROUGH RELAPSE-PREVENTION STRATEGIES WITH THIS STRESSOR IN MIND, WRITING DOWN CLIENT-GENERATED IDEAS IN ADDITION TO THE ONES PROVIDED].

*Awesome. That sounds like a good plan. Now, Tess, the other piece I have been wondering about is that we talked about how your mother has been unhappy both about your decision to pursue graduate school instead of entering the workforce and even about you coming into therapy. I know both of those have gotten somewhat better with some of the efforts we have made in therapy to talk about both. I'm just curious, are there any other situations you expect where you might receive some pushback on using the skills we have learned here, or toward your vocational choices because it might be in conflict with the main cultural or societal beliefs surrounding you? What do you think you can do if those situations arise, based on what we learned here, so you don't stop doing the activities that bring you the most joy and well-being and still respect the beliefs of those important to you?*

[GUIDELINE 5: Addressing stigma and other cultural barriers in treatment]

**Tess**: *Well, I actually think my dad would be okay with it if he is able to come here soon. My brothers are just young so they may not understand. I think I can talk openly about why I want to go to graduate school and use ways to manage my stress, and this might actually be a good model for my brothers. In fact, I'm more worried about this guy I have started dating recently that I mentioned before. He is also Latino, but he is born and raised here, so I don't really know how he feels about the therapy piece in particular. I know he knows I get stressed out, but we have never talked about it, because I don't want to scare him off. I guess if I'm scared to do it, I should probably raise it, huh? [laughs]*

**Therapist** [smiling]: *Yup, you got it. Good takeaway from what we learned here! But let's brainstorm together how you may broach the topic, and deal with any negative feedback you may get from him about your mental health. We can write it down so you don't have to necessarily come up with it completely spontaneously—even though you know I think it's good to become comfortable with some uncertainty! But maybe just some general points you can have in mind.* [LEADS CLIENT THROUGH THIS BRIEFLY].

*Wonderful, Tess. You have some great things in place to make sure you keep your skills up and manage your anxiety even way after therapy is over. One last thing I have had on my mind is what we have talked about in terms of your future job prospects, and dealing with discrimination or microaggressions from others about your immigration status. I know we have dealt with that a good deal during therapy, but what ideas do you have around what specific skills you can use to either challenge your anxious thoughts, approach a situation you're avoiding (like applying for jobs!), engage in good self-care, or seek the advocates or other help to support you in directly addressing discriminatory actions by others? I want to help you have a clear plan in place if this occurs again, and also give you a space here to discuss what worries you about these possibilities so we can come up with some constructive ways to help you cope with this and get everything you rightly deserve, as unfair and maddening as such treatment is likely to be.*

[GUIDELINE 6: Exploring the impact of discrimination and micro-aggressions on therapy]

[LEADS CLIENT THROUGH THIS REFLECTION AND ADDS TO THE RELAPSE PREVENTION].

*Excellent, Tess, I'm so impressed by how well you're able to apply what you found helpful in our time together to think ahead about what might be stressful or upsetting in the future so you have a plan. What are we missing that we want to plan ahead for, or that you'd love some guidance on how to tackle for the future?*

*Summary of guideline application.* Obviously, it will not always be necessary or possible to use all seven guidelines when doing relapse prevention planning, and that is completely fine. Here the therapist chooses the top ones that they feel are most important to touch on based on their relationship with the client and what have come up as most salient for Tess over the course of therapy. And one guideline that permeates throughout this discussion is the cultural humility practice in Guideline 2, as the therapist takes an open, non-judgmental, and partnered approach with her client to figuring out the best way to proceed and what they should be thinking about together.

When you do your own reflection using Exercise 8.1, it is simply to ensure that you have considered all the guidelines to provide culturally responsive treatment through this important phase of relapse-prevention planning, given the importance of this phase in most evidence-based protocols to prevent relapse and return of symptoms, so we can keep our clients as well as we can for as long as possible.

Exercise 8.1

CHECKLIST OF GUIDELINES FOR RELAPSE-PREVENTION TREATMENT PLANNING

Use this list to jot down which guidelines may be relevant and what points specific to your client you might want to raise for each. For guidelines that are not relevant or not high priority to touch on, simply indicate N/A, but a general rule of thumb is that 2–3 guidelines are likely highly applicable to your client.

**Guideline 1: Exploring Your Own Cultural Identity, Beliefs, and Biases Before Providing Therapy**

_____

_____

_____

**Guideline 2: Practicing Cultural Humility as a Continuous Process**

_____

_____

_____

**Guideline 3: Balancing Culturally Informed and Individualized Assessment of the Presenting Problem**

_____

_____

_____

**Guideline 4: Engaging in Self-Education about Specific Cultural Norms Using a Variety of Sources**

_____

_____

_____

**Guideline 5: Addressing Stigma and Other Cultural Barriers to Psychological Treatment**

_____

_____

_____

**Guideline 6: Exploring the Impact of Discrimination and Microaggressions on Therapy**

_____

_____

_____

**Guideline 7: Identifying and Incorporating Cultural Strengths and Resources into Treatment**

_____

_____

_____

_____

## COMMENTARY ON INCORPORATING SOCIAL JUSTICE

Something that continues to concern me as a clinician, health disparities researcher, and community advocate is how to deliver treatments that not only make a wider swath of our community better, but also *keep* them well for longer. To this end, I think the importance of incorporating and utilizing identity-based facets into relapse-prevention and treatment-summary processes often falls by the wayside, and I think this is a disservice to those we pledge to help. When we commit to incorporating diversity considerations and to partner with our clients throughout the entire treatment process, we are making a commitment to empower them to take the evidence-based strategies we teach them during treatment into their everyday lives long after therapy is over. Given that this is the aim of any relapse-prevention efforts, how can we not spend the time to make sure such strategies are effectively and consistently woven into their own unique life fabric? By making this effort in our final treatment sessions, we are acknowledging that even the best strategies have limits in their effectiveness if they are not congruent with the rich, varied lives our clients want to have, and in this way we engage in socially just and culturally competent clinical practice.

## SUMMARY

All in all, what you have hopefully ensured with your client by repeated use of the guidelines throughout treatment at this final stage of treatment is an open dialogue about the ways their identity factors intersect with their mental health concerns. Keeping the impact of our intersectional identity facets on all experiences of life (including our emotional health) at the forefront will allow you to think about how this will continue to be the case even after your time with your client is over. With this appreciation, and through the open lines of communication about identity issues that you have established with your client, you and your client will be well positioned to effectively complete relapse-prevention planning and give them the best shot at maintaining their important gains from your time together.

# 9

# Considerations for the Supervisory Relationship with Diverse Trainees and Their Diverse Clients

The last area I want to spend some time on is supervision. Specifically, I have been asked by a number of clinics and training programs to address the practice of culturally competent supervision, which has some overlap with, but some distinctly unique issues from, culturally competent clinical care. Luckily, the guidelines I present can be applied to this domain, but I thought it would be useful to clearly delineate how they should be considered (and practiced) within the supervisor-supervisee relationship, *particularly* as they relate to supervising trainees who are themselves from diverse, underrepresented backgrounds in psychology.

To this point, as someone who has been a supervisee/trainee of color for many years and who is now a supervisor, considering what comes up for our supervisees who are from any number of diverse identities based on race, gender identity, sexual orientation, disability status, age, income level, etc., was a particularly important chapter for me to write. Even beyond my personal reasons and interest in exploring this, we have a growing appreciation for how truly diverse our trainees are, which is a great development for our field, particularly in terms of building capacity within our communities to better address ongoing health disparities (Commission on Accreditation, 2020; Duan, 2020). In addition, our students themselves are pushing for us to consider issues of diversity more significantly in our provision of training (Gregus, Stevens, Seivert, Tucker, & Callahan, 2019; Lee & Khawaja, 2013). Given these factors, I was puzzled by the lack of data in the literature about the unique challenges faced by our supervisees in terms of their identity characteristics (and particularly when these differ saliently from their supervisors), and limited published guidance on how to address issues of discrimination, microaggressions, and identity-based conflict that are likely to arise in supervisory situations as we all work toward diversifying our trainee pool on multiple identity facets.

*A Cultural Humility and Social Justice Approach to Psychotherapy.* Anu Asnaani, Oxford University Press.
© Oxford University Press 2023. DOI: 10.1093/oso/9780197635971.003.0010

The few articles that do examine this area have found several consistent themes. First, there is documented bias in clinical supervision and teaching, for instance with long-standing perpetuation of heterosexual norms (Pilkington & Cantor, 1996), although this has started to at least generate some dialogue about working with trainees of diverse gender and sexual identities (e.g., Pfohl, 2004; Halpert & Pfaller, 2001). And certainly such bias has been documented around re-peated discrimination and microaggressions committed toward trainees of color occurring within supervision (e.g., Constantine & Sue, 2007). The published lit-erature, however, does not currently focus on the conflict that could arise from any other number of identity differences that are likely to occur in supervision, even though we contemporarily encounter these other important identity aspects (e.g., working with trainees with visible or invisible disabilities, international trainees, first-generation college/graduate school trainees who are simultaneously navigating the experience of graduate school with their clinical training, among many others). Taken together, these findings and observations highlight the dire need for the supervisor to demonstrate a high level of cultural competence within the supervisory relationship.

Colleagues in social work have offered some important models and spe-cific practices to consider to achieve cultural competency within supervision. For instance, Lipscomb and Ashley (2017) utilize case studies, ethnographic observations of the authors' own supervision experiences, and interviews with supervisors and supervisees to better understand their perspectives on crucial aspects related to identity in the supervision context, including impacts of power, privilege, and race within the supervisory dyad. Importantly, they highlight the utility of concepts we have already raised in this book for supervision, including cultural sensitivity, cultural humility, and modeling of authentic responding as supervisors. They also provide practical strategies for supervisors to approach difficult topics about identity with their trainees (which I also offer in Box 9.1) and other practical recommendations to create a culturally competent supervi-sion context. Another article, while it is a case study by the author based on her own experiences with two specific positive supervisory interactions as a Black fe-male trainee (Gómez, 2020), provides rich insight into the ways we can empower our supervisees to address issues of identity, discrimination, and their own lived experiences within supervision, closely mirroring the strategies for supervisors to consider as outlined by Lipscomb and Ashley (2017). There is also an illuminating chapter that provides additional guidance around navigating issues of diversity in supervision, and which further highlights how such efforts are in line with both culturally competent teaching and socially just practice, as such efforts promote mental health equity and address intersectional issues of power that arise within the supervision context (Oshin, Ching, & West, 2019).

Still, given the dearth of published material on this area and the lack of study in clinical psychology in particular, I have to admit that in this chapter I some-what have to wade into guidance that is more based on my own professional experiences as a supervisor and as a trainee, guidance that is not as rooted in the published literature or corroborated by experts in the field as I typically prefer

Box 9.1

## Sample Prompts to Address Instances Where You Have Committed a Microaggression toward Your Supervisee within the Context of Supervision

If you are aware that you have committed a microaggression toward your supervisee, well done. This is half the battle, and now it's time to fix the misstep and to try to preserve the clinical supervision relationship. Remember your core values, and be brave to accept fault, regardless of the power differential that exists. And as always, this list gives you some ideas of how to raise the issue, but certainly consult with colleagues where you can, to get additional support, guidance, and ideas. Remember, by raising your own missteps with supervisees, you are modeling cultural humility for their own training, while simultaneously engaging in an act of social justice to reduce the disparities and disproportionately poorer treatment faced by supervisees from underrepresented backgrounds.

Sample prompts to bring this up in your supervision meeting or to explore whether such microaggressions have occurred without your awareness:

* *X, before we get started with reviewing your clients today, I just wanted to raise something that happened last week that has been on my mind. Specifically, I want to apologize for when I said/did XYZ* [**be explicit about what it was! Don't be vague**] *last week, and I am sorry if that was hurtful to you. I have been doing my own reflection about my values as a supervisor, and I realize that I have some of my own biases or preconceived notions about clinical supervision that might have clouded the way I treated you. This is not fair to you, and I am truly sorry for that.*

* *As your clinical supervisor, I am here to support you and provide the best training I can to you. It is my intention to always strive to provide the most open, accepting, and safe environment for you to reach your training goals, and by doing XYZ* [**be explicit, no excuses!**], *I violated that promise of such a safe space. That is not in line with my professional values, and I am truly sorry that I behaved in such a way. I felt* [**shame, guilt, anger at myself, sadness, etc.**] *by how I behaved/what I said.*

* *Would you be open to sharing how you felt or what you thought when I said/did XYZ? What was that like for you?*

* *I am working hard on my own self-reflection about when I commit behaviors that are unacceptable or unfair to you, but I would love to create a space where you feel comfortable letting me know when I inadvertently act in similar ways or am offensive to you. What are some ways I can make you feel like this is a professional relationship where you can raise those types of concerns?*

* *Are there any other instances of mistreatment or biased behavior from your perspective that we haven't talked about that you are comfortable bringing up right now? It's totally okay if there isn't, I know I have some work to do to make you trust that this is a safe space to discuss such issues within our supervision relationship. But if you have anything to raise while we are discussing it today, I'm all ears.*

and as is the default for the rest of the material in this book. Still, the issue is too important to simply omit, and in general, much of the specific guidance of navigating issues of difference with our supervisees is fairly consistent with how we think about addressing identity-related differences even with our clients (for whom we do have considerably more guidance from the field). I therefore rely on the guidelines I have already outlined in previous chapters, and in the next section I have tried to extrapolate from these to demonstrate how they may apply to the supervisory context. This is by no means an exhaustive application of culturally competent guidelines for clinical supervision, and I encourage all supervisors to think about how any of the guidelines in this book may be relevant to your responsibility as a trainer of the next generation of therapists. I end by providing a few brief exercises and figures that serve as shorthand guides to addressing any identity-based ruptures that may occur in the supervisor-supervisee relationship, and some brief commentary on how such approaches align with a social justice mindset.

## INCORPORATING OUR GUIDELINES INTO SUPERVISION WITH DIVERSE SUPERVISEES

When thinking about providing supervision either to supervisees who themselves identify with an intersection of diverse identities, or who are providing care to clients from a variety of intersecting identities (or both), several of the guidelines are likely to be particularly helpful. First, I cannot stress enough how important it is when we are wearing our supervisor hats to engage in continuous, deep, and authentic reflection about our own cultural identities, and the beliefs/biases we bring to the domain of clinical care *and* clinical training of others. A common misstep I hear from others (and have experienced firsthand) is a false sense of security that we have reached a stage of "cultural actualization" as supervisors based on our own identities or experience working with a range of clients, and that we can, therefore, not be biased or possibly perpetuate unfair treatment of our trainees. Nothing could be further from the truth! Guideline 1 (exploring our own identities, biases, and beliefs) thus becomes central to our own roles as supervisors, regardless of our own individual identities. Specifically, what are we aware of, in terms of our own comfort zones and internal thoughts, feelings, and behavioral tendencies, when we are working with a supervisee from clearly different identity markers than our own, or who is bringing forth a client from a background identity for which we already hold preconceived beliefs or biases? What self-reflection and work do we want to apply from Guideline 1 in the domain of providing clinical supervision?

Similarly, Guideline 2 (practicing cultural humility) goes hand in hand with such a self-reflection. How do we show our willingness to continuously learn and be open to making missteps with our supervisees in our feedback to them, or when referring to their diverse clients? The exercises and strategies to build cultural humility in Guideline 2 can be translated to our work as supervisors. Again, it is important to remember that none of us is immune to such cultural missteps; in fact, others have explored the very idea that supervisors who are themselves from diverse identity backgrounds can perpetuate the same microaggressive or biased behaviors that we want to safeguard our supervisees from (Jernigan, Green, Helms, Perez-Gualdron, & Henze, 2010; Murphy-Shigematsu, 2010). I occasionally encounter the idea that my teaching on cultural competency in supervision is only meant for our White colleagues; this both reduces the many multifaceted and rich aspects of identity to one (race), and ignores the fact that this skill applies to each and every one of us.

To consolidate the main teachings of Guidelines 1 and 2 into the context of supervision, Exercise 9.1 provides a worksheet for supervisors to assess our own power, privilege, and biases in the context of clinical supervision, and to take stock of where we may need to do more of our reflection or active alliance-building with our supervisees. You can always revisit Chapter 2 on cultural humility to brush up on other ways to practice humility when you recognize that you have made a misstep or have engaged in a biased behavior toward your trainee, but to distill the main idea here: in short, we have to be open to actively modeling how to share our own missteps, and importantly, demonstrate how we hold ourselves accountable for these errors in practice (either with our own clients, or with our supervisees). Similarly, we need to be mindful about actively demonstrating our own cultural competency; for example, offering our own pronouns within the context of group or individual supervision, avoiding stereotypical characterizations of clients, and reminding supervisees to consider intersectional identity factors that may be at play for the clients they treat. In this way, we show our trainees how to practice cultural humility more broadly for all clients served, even when they do not automatically raise these issues in regard to specific clients.

Exercise 9.1

## SUPERVISOR REFLECTION OF POWER, PRIVILEGE, AND BIASES TOWARD SUPERVISEES

Think about the following questions as they relate specifically to your supervisee. Answer as honestly and openly as you can, to fully understand which aspects might potentially facilitate or hinder the ideal working relationship in clinical supervision.

1. **Reflection on identity and power/privilege differentials between you and your supervisee**:

a. What are some of the salient identity differences and similarities you believe you share with your supervisee? Think broadly about identity on multiple facets of one's identity (e.g., anchoring back to the ADDRESSING model by Hays, 2022).

**Differences in identity**: _____

**Similarities in identity**: _____

b. How about in terms of the power and privilege you hold as a supervisor? How does this further intersect with these identity differences and/or similarities?

i. **Nature of the power differential between me and my supervisee**:

_____

**This could impact our working relationship in the following ways**:

_____

ii. **Nature of the privilege differential between me and my supervisee**:

_____

**This could impact our working relationship in the following ways**:

_____

2. **Reflection on your own biases as a supervisor or specifically in terms of salient identity markers for your supervisee:**

a. What negative judgments have I noticed I make about my supervisees based on a range of factors (their level of training, type of training, or a host of identity markers such as race, gender, sexual orientation, religion, etc.)?

_____

_____

b. Have I noticed that any of these negative thoughts/judgments come up in the context of working with this particular supervisee?

_____

_____

c. Being honest with myself, have I observed that these negative beliefs have impacted the way I have treated my supervisee or how I have engaged with them in the context of clinical supervision? Be specific here about what these behaviors have been.

_____

_____

d. Having written down the ways I may have behaved in biased ways with my trainee, how do I feel about it? How is this behavior in line or in contrast with my core values as a supervisor?

_____

_____

_____

In addition, Guideline 6 (exploring the impact of discrimination and microaggressions in therapy) plays a large role within the realm of culturally competent clinical supervision. As noted earlier, a number of studies have shown that microaggressions commonly occur within the supervisory context, often perpetuated toward trainees of color or other underrepresented identities in psychology (Constantine & Sue, 2007; Hernández & McDowell, 2010). It is paramount, therefore, that as supervisors we are aware of when we commit such microaggressions toward our trainees and work actively to address these gross missteps and maltreatment. Many of the exercises and figures in Chapter 6 can assist in this effort and can be applied across clinical therapy and clinical supervision situations. However, given the differences in the relationship we share with our supervisees versus our clients, the ways in which we raise such instances where we have engaged in discrimination or microaggressions with our supervisees are nuanced and specific to this professional dynamic. In Box 9.1, I try to provide some sample prompts that we can utilize as supervisors to raise such ruptures in the supervisory relationship with our trainees. Importantly, if you are aware that you have committed a microaggression toward your supervisee, please also review Chapter 6 on addressing discrimination perpetuated in therapy, as many of the concepts, worksheets, and skills will relate to managing this same area within clinical supervision.

## WHAT IF I AM THE SUPERVISEE WHO HAS BEEN MISTREATED?

From the opposite perspective, it may be that you are a supervisee from any number of underrepresented backgrounds, and that you have experienced unfair or biased treatment from your supervisor. This is a tricky situation because of the professional and evaluative nature of one's relationship with their supervisor, and the inherent power/privilege differentials that exist, as we explored earlier. Regardless of any of these, if you are a supervisee who has been mistreated based on your own identity factors, you are completely justified in ensuring that this unfair and, frankly, unethical treatment is stopped or addressed immediately. In Box 9.2, I provide some tips for the ways in which you can obtain the support and assistance in pushing your supervisor to stop this behavior, which include whom you can initially approach for support (e.g., another faculty member in your training area, a senior colleague, or colleagues from outside your institution), and then whom you can go to next to raise the alarm at a higher level (e.g., another supervisor on the team or team/clinic lead).

Importantly, I think it is crucial as one of the bigger objectives in your own professional development training that you at least consider raising the issue directly with your supervisor if it feels safe enough to do so after consulting with your initial level of support, if you don't share a rapport with your supervisor where you can immediately do so. In this regard, I provide some sample prompts for how you may raise the issue directly with your supervisor; you are warned that some

Box 9.2

SAMPLE PROMPTS TO RAISE INSTANCES OF MICROAGGRESSIONS OR BIASED TREATMENT AIMED TOWARD YOU AS A TRAINEE, PERPETUATED BY YOUR SUPERVISOR

It can be really hard to raise issues of mistreatment when you're on the receiving end of it, and particularly with someone who inherently holds power over your training and part of your professional trajectory. While we all hope that supervisors will themselves raise the issues, some are unwilling, but many are also unaware that they have engaged in behavior that is biased or microaggressive. Don't automatically assume a negative intention by your supervisor; check your own experiences that may be categorizing your supervisor as someone else who has been intentionally discriminatory, and see if you can approach the situation with an openness and with compassion. And what if after attempting to address the issue with your supervisor, it doesn't work? Well, then it's time to get the support you deserve elsewhere, as outlined after these sample prompts for first trying to raise the issue directly with your supervisor.

Sample prompts to bring up an instance of biased behavior by your supervisor or general feelings of being dismissed or unfairly treated (ideally in an individual meeting with your supervisor to reduce defensiveness by your supervisor, if this feels safe to do so):

* *X, before we get started with reviewing my clients today, I just wanted to raise something that happened last week that has been on my mind. Specifically, I wanted to share that when you said/did XYZ* [**be as explicit as you can, so there is no confusion about what occurred**] *last week, I felt* [**anger, sadness, disappointment, surprise, etc.**] *because this felt like unfair treatment* **OR** *that I was being singled out based on my XX identity* **OR** *it didn't take my XX identity facet into account, and that felt disrespectful/ disappointing. Can we spend some of our supervision time today talking about that some more?*

* *I want to get the most out of supervision with you, and while our focus is on providing the best clinical care to my clients that you supervise, when these types of interactions occur between you and me, it makes me feel less able to do that or engage in our clinical supervision to my full capacity. I would like to talk about how we can discuss differences between us in terms of our backgrounds or perspectives about therapy so that we can be respectful of each other's perspectives and get the most out of supervision. Would this be possible to spend some time doing this? It's important to me.*

* [If this feels safe and authentic to do] *I have faced a lot of discrimination over my lifetime in other personal and professional contexts, particularly directed toward* [name specific or intersectional identity facets here], *and it has been a challenge for me to experience similar dynamics here. I want to be able to have a supervision relationship where we can discuss these issues and I can raise these experiences if they occur in supervision with you without a fear of being dismissed or those experiences being minimized. I would value having such an open dialogue with you, and I think it would be great for both our professional relationship and in terms of my broader training.*

In sum, you can raise your own feelings about what specific instances or features of your interaction with your supervisor feel discriminatory or biased, while still stating an intention to build a strong working alliance and training relationship with them.

But what if they are not responsive, become defensive, or dismiss your concerns as unimportant? If you have given it a try to raise this directly with your supervisor, here are some others you can go to, depending on your comfort level and specific interpersonal/department/training clinic dynamics. Note, each will have different levels of support they can provide, from informal suggestions or guidance of what to do next, to disciplinary ability. A good rule of thumb is to start with someone who can provide more support and a listening ear about best next steps, who may provide a few more suggestions of how to address the issue again with your supervisor, or who may alternatively advise you to immediately "dial up" your report of this behavior, because of a standing pattern of mistreatment or due to the egregiousness of it. That next level of outreach typically can help you come to a more formal resolution or administrative-level intervention.

Initial
* Senior trainee/colleague
* Another faculty member in your training area
* External colleagues/scholars/mentors (not at your training setting or institution)

Next Steps
* Another supervisor on your team
* Director of clinical training/clinic director

supervisors (depending on their own levels of cultural competency and humility) may not be able to constructively receive your feedback. In this case, following some of the other ways to obtain support from others to encourage a chance in communication may prove more fruitful, particularly those higher levels of support that I outline as "next steps" in Box 9.2. Nonetheless, I encourage you to first raise the rupture with your supervisor to try to come to a resolution with them directly if they do not raise it first (and again, only if it seems safe and appropriate to do so).

## SUMMARY AND COMMENTARY ON INCORPORATING SOCIAL JUSTICE

One remaining area I want to pre-emptively address within the supervision domain is how we can ensure our regular (and required) constructive feedback to our trainees is not simply categorized as microaggressive or discriminatory by our trainees. That is, what do we say to those who (validly) raise the concern that if we open the floor to our trainees to raise any grievances they have in our interaction style or supervision content, we will handicap our own ability to provide any kind of constructive feedback without it being chalked up to us being culturally insensitive or biased? Again, in the absence of much-needed academic and published debate about this, I can only share what colleagues and I have raised in conversation and my own take on this question. By the way, I would note that this is not just a concern for supervision, but also for doing culturally competent evidence-based practice (EBP) more broadly. Specifically, detractors of the push for improving our cultural competency have offered the same concern, i.e., that we threaten the core, active ingredients of EBP by making *too* many cultural modifications or accommodations. In other words, conducting culturally competent and socially just therapy sacrifices the very elements that make our EBPs useful and effective.

My counterargument to both of these similar critiques for supervision or practice is largely the same: while these are indeed possibilities (rare, from my experience), the harm we stand to inflict upon our trainees (or clients) by *not* raising these issues of identity in our work (and the probability of such harm occurring, per documented instances) is much higher than the chance that we will prioritize cultural competency approaches or advocate for fair treatment of others to the exclusion of good supervision (or practice). And the solution for both is the same: open and transparent communication. Talking with our trainees directly about whether the identity differences are overshadowing the provision of good supervisory guidance (if this indeed occurs) is the best course of action we have to address this situation. This includes a validation of the concerns around identity differences, with a clear statement of our commitment to providing good supervision while providing a safe space for our supervisees to raise issues that directly impact their own sense of well-being and efficacy. Isn't this the balance we are charged with anyway as supervisors, clinical instructors, and teachers? From a social justice perspective, I emphatically agree with colleagues who reiterate that this is our burden as supervisors to bear—to fight hard to find that balance (Hair, 2015). Our supervisees have had enough of their own challenges based on their identities and have their own challenges to navigate with clients in this regard. It is our primary responsibility as supervisors to create this safe, culturally humble, open, and helpful space to facilitate our trainees' growth and progress.

# 10

# Final Thoughts

As this book draws to a close, I wanted to share a few final thoughts about my own journey toward cultural humility and social justice, and lessons I have learned so far, in my last dedicated space to do so.

The first set of thoughts are practical in nature, and continue from the guidelines, strategies, and tips that have been the central focus of this book. For instance, I want to acknowledge that in this book I did not explore in any depth the specific cultural modifications to evidence-based practices (EBPs) that may exist (and have been tested) for specific disorders in specific populations. This does not mean that such practices do not exist; they very much do, and our field has greatly benefited from many visionaries who have worked tirelessly in the health disparities arena of mental health to propose and subsequently adequately test such culturally responsive treatment protocols (see the references in the Appendix for some examples for specific identity groups and some great resources, such as work by Zane and colleagues, among many others; Zane, Bernal, & Leong, 2016). Further, while there are undoubtedly (and unfortunately) fewer studies that have examined such cultural modifications to EBPs (Rathod et al., 2018), we do know from meta-analytic examinations that have pooled these studies' findings that, in general, treatments that have been modified to be culturally responsive tend to outperform those that are not modified with diversity considerations in mind (Griner & Smith, 2006; Soto, Smith, Griner, Rodriguez, & Bernal, 2019).

Thus, while I did not specifically mention this in the guidelines, let me take a chance to do so here: when confronted with a client with a particular identity (or intersection of identities, as is more likely the case), it would be prudent for us as therapists who value empirical findings and scientific examination to refer back to the literature for any specific treatment recommendations for the psychological symptoms at hand in the specific identity categories of the client in question (Asnaani & Hofmann, 2012). Consistent with much of our academic training, we would (1) rely on any larger trials of the culturally modified treatment (if it exists); (2) consider single case studies when larger studies don't exist (or in addition); and then (3) refer to published clinical guidelines from experts in the field who can distill some of their experience with specific groups into theoretical models or guidelines to advise our own work. Following this attempt to

*A Cultural Humility and Social Justice Approach to Psychotherapy.* Anu Asnaani, Oxford University Press.
© Oxford University Press 2023. DOI: 10.1093/oso/9780197635971.003.0011

utilize our pooled knowledge as a field, (4) Guideline 4 (considering a full range of sources for cultural knowledge) could then be utilized to further inform our own cultural modifications/additions, with sole reliance on this method of culturally informing our treatment approach only in the *absence* of any existing literature or prior work relevant to the specific case we are treating.

For instance, in keeping with social justice principles and our acknowledgment of social determinants of health, we might need to supplement our treatments with other strategies to ensure validity and maximum impact of our EBP. This might include providing assistance on adding financial or vocational services, or helping clients get connected to language, employment, or educational services. It might also entail connecting clients to trusted surrogates in the community who can help them navigate the unique challenges they may face based on any one of their intersectional identity factors (e.g., ensuring that our clients from the LGBTQIA+ community have an advocate who can help keep them safe and supported if they encounter discrimination in the workplace or even while trying to engage in therapy homework in public settings; Hope et al., 2022). In addition, as alluded to in several of our guidelines, it's important to consider the *context* in which your client is operating, to better account for how your treatment may need to be modified or supplemented for maximum effectiveness. For instance, is your client living in poverty in an otherwise affluent area, or are they one of the few immigrants in the town in which they live and work? Not all modifications are equal and warranted without taking into account these immediate considerations and intersections of identity with the broader societal context.

The second area I want to address is how these guidelines for culturally competent clinical practice relate to good health disparities research, which is my main area of scientific inquiry outside of the work I do as a therapist, supervisor, and trainer (although, one may argue, an area that is directly connected to all my professional roles). It has been fascinating to me that in the over 15 years that I have been deeply steeped in the field of clinical psychological science, very few individuals have questioned my clinical approach to integrating diversity considerations into EBP (and I have been very appreciative of those who have been critical, in my continued quest to improve my own cultural competency). Yet, as someone who holds a strong academic and research focus, a badge of honor worn as a central element of my professional identity, I *have* received considerable criticism about my research work in assessing, proposing, and testing cultural modifications to EBP. Those critical of my work have provided feedback closely mirroring the idea that proposing cultural modifications and testing such adaptations to existing EBPs are simply examining the impact of "window-dressing" of an already efficacious treatment, and such pursuits are somehow elementary or superficial in their potential impacts. Specifically, the undertone of such opposition to this line of my (and many of my esteemed colleagues') work is that we know that these treatments work, and now clinicians should be left to do what good therapists do, i.e., make that effective treatment acceptable to a client from a particular intersection of identities that may not have been included in the original efficacy data of the treatment to begin with. It is likely not a surprise to you that I disagree strongly with this sentiment, and I think it's a harmful perspective to be so dismissive about the importance of real cultural adaptations of a treatment.

I say this as a person whose main line of work within addressing health disparities is not just to see if "established" treatments work for a wider diversity of individuals, but to understand how and why they work (and don't work). For instance, I have particular interest in understanding the potential mechanisms of empirically supported treatments (ESTs)—do they result in symptom reduction because the active ingredients directly target the symptoms, or do they work via an intermediary variable like emotion regulation, tolerance to distress, or even specific cultural value orientations or group-specific conceptualizations of mental health? Thus, I see the work to propose and test cultural adaptations to ESTs as multilevel examinations of the mechanisms that may act differently based on one's intersectional identities (not just based on the disorder symptoms we are trying to target). Such an approach also begs the question of whether we actually need to throw out the playbook on the way to study a particular disorder/treatment altogether and create a new treatment that is culturally responsive from its inception, using more rigorous diversity science approaches (Lau, Chang, & Okazaki, 2010). This is a tension that continues to exist due to the conflict for some scholars between engaging in EBP and taking a culturally humble/socially just approach, which has been highlighted as potentially incongruent with one another (Sue, Sue, Neville, & Smith, 2022). Or, maybe we actually need to focus our efforts on empowering communities to reclaim traditional forms of healing that already exist in their cultural contexts, which we have diminished or dismissed from a Western perspective—another idea that other scholars in the field have rightly suggested may be the case for many underserved communities (e.g., Gone, 2021).

That said, this book has focused on what we can do with the treatments we know to be effective right now, those with an evidence base that make us feel more confident in utilizing a specific treatment approach for a particular set of symptoms (at least until more compelling evidence arises). My own (and admittedly biased) perspective on the tension between "evidence-based" and "culturally responsive" is that these two elements are not divergent, and that just as we don't know with complete certainty that our current EBPs work with diverse populations because of a lack of inclusion of diverse clients in the initial testing of such treatments, we also don't know that these treatments *won't* work just because the identity factors of a particular client presenting to us for treatment are different from those included in the larger clinical research. And for this reason, I return to how published literature has guided the recommendations I made in this book at a broader level, with one overarching consistent message across the field being clear: regardless where you stand on the evidence-based versus culturally responsive treatment spectrum, the relationship shared between the client and the therapist matters. And I say this as a die-hard CBT clinician and researcher, who has engaged in academic debate about this idea that therapeutic alliance and other common factors of therapy do not matter as much as the effective, "active" ingredients of a treatment (e.g., see my impassioned commentary speaking to the same in Asnaani & Foa, 2015). Yet, I cannot deny the assertions of my highly knowledgeable colleagues who specialize in cross-cultural mental health work, coupled with my own observations as a clinician and supervisor with diverse clients, that none of our EBPs matter if a client doesn't feel heard and respected for who they are as a person. As a result, the guidelines I have put forth in this book are aimed at strengthening that very therapeutic alliance that I have questioned the utility of as a researcher. I have to own this seeming contradiction in my clinical versus research work, and this is a discrepancy I am still trying to reconcile as I continue to grow within my own research and practice.

Finally, the last area I want to touch on is more philosophical and personal in nature. I started this book with full transparency about my own intersectional identity markers and unique life and professional experiences that have framed the way I think about culturally competent and culturally humble practice. This is very similar to how I start my in-person trainings on this same topic. As I mentioned in the Introduction of this book, I believe that such openness about possible beliefs (and biases) based on these intersectional factors is crucial to have at the forefront of such discussions. Why? Because I see such disclosure as a meta-model for how we should approach therapy with each of our clients to begin with, to ensure we bring our most authentic selves to the therapy process.

Specifically, as a person of color, as an immigrant, as a parent, as a cis-gendered woman, and as a health disparities researcher, I hold the values of authenticity and social justice/fairness as central to how I live my life across the many roles I have. To be clear, I do not expect others to espouse these same values, and charging mental health professionals to engage in social justice has not been without its controversy or resistance (Ali & Sichel, 2019). These values are simply the ones I have used as my own guide to my work and identity in the field (and in the world, in general). As a result, this book reflects my own desire to produce work in line with those core values that I hold dear. This book is also a concerted attempt to collate and share the knowledge of our many exceptional scholars in the field, integrated with my own clinical experience over the past decade and a half of clinical practice, as they are framed by my own values-based lens. Take from it what you will for your own practice, and I only hope some of the guidance from this book can empower you to continue to act in line with your own professional and personal values.

# ACKNOWLEDGMENTS

This work would not be possible without the direction, opportunities provided to me, and advocacy from a number of individuals I have been beyond fortunate to have in my corner. First, I want to thank my graduate school mentor, Dr. Stefan Hofmann, who first presented the idea of examining the topic of culturally competent evidence-based therapy to me as an advanced graduate student over a decade ago and let me take the lead on an invited paper on the topic, which ended up serving as a launching point for all of my subsequent work in this area. As is true of so many of my career directions, Stefan provided the push for me to fly, and he exuded trust in me that my wings would carry me, and for that I'm very grateful to him. I am also extremely thankful for Sarah Harrington, my editor at Oxford University Press, who spotted my work at a conference some six years ago and saw something that told her that I had an important contribution to make, and encouraged me to pursue such a project to share my work with others in the field. She has been an unbelievable advocate and support, without whom I would not have persisted in such an endeavor. In addition, I am full of gratitude to Dr. Pamela Hays, who not only kindly agreed to provide a Foreword for this current book, but also has been such a supportive and cherished colleague given her own immense scholarship in this field. She embodies humility and generosity, and she has provided such warm positive regard that I have been honored to receive given her immense stature as an expert in the cross-cultural psychology field.

Aside from the professional direction and support, there is absolutely no way I would be able to produce this work without my broader support network over the past decade. From my parents, who highlighted cross-cultural issues by being immigrants themselves in a foreign land and trying to instill pride in me for both our native and adopted cultures, to my extended family and dear friends throughout my life from all over the world who have showed me the value and richness of a diversity of cultures firsthand, to communities who have trusted me to partner with them to address health disparities and generously shared with me their own culturally informed conceptions of mental health, I am often in awe of how lucky I am to have had such experiences uniquely shape my own view of health, well-being, and thriving.

Of course, most proximal to this book is the influence, support, and encouragement of my husband, Peter, and the patience/tolerance of my absence in the hours spent to write the book by my now preschool-aged daughter Neena, without both of whom I would have never even embarked on such a project. Raising our daughter in a German–St. Lucian–Indian–American household, where we try to embody values and practices from all four (quite disparate) cultures, has been in equal measure fairly challenging, wildly interesting, intensely fun, and immensely instructional to my own identity as a psychologist. I can't count my blessings enough for having Peter as an equal, loving life partner and Neena as an active (and vocal!) participant in this juggling act.

Finally, this work signifies both an end and a beginning. First, it is the culmination of years of research, scholarship, training, clinical experience, and teaching from so many insightful and brilliant scholars, colleagues, and trainees in the field who have pushed me to expand my own understanding of diversity, inclusion, and equity as these concepts relate to culturally competent and socially just clinical practice through their own immense work and contributions to this topic. For each of these individuals and what they have taught me, I am so very thankful.

On the other hand, this book also marks a new beginning for me professionally; it has put into writing a commitment to socially just clinical practice (and by extension, my research and training/teaching). It is my public declaration that this is an area that will continue to be central to all my future pursuits in the field. Consequently, it also opens the flood gates for scrutiny if I ever fall short of these ideals of social justice and cultural humility in my roles as a clinical psychologist. However, I am proud to continue to strive to exemplify these ideals in all aspects of my work, and to be transparent in my efforts (and likely occasional failures) to do so, including being ready to accept the critiques of this book itself where it falls short in this effort. And for that ability to be open to failure, to learn, to course correct, and to grow, I am thankful for those parts of my own life journey (the lows and the highs) that have brought me here and will take me onward.

Exercises

The exercises provided in *A Cultural Humility and Social Justice Approach to Psychotherapy: Seven Applied Guidelines for Evidence-Based Practice* can also be accessed online by searching for this book's title on the Oxford Academic platform, at academic.oup.com.

Exercise 1.1

## Self-Identification Worksheet

| Identity Factor | How Others Identify Me | How I Identify |
|---|---|---|
| Age and generational influences | | |
| Developmental disabilities | | |
| Disabilities (other) | | |
| Religion and spirituality | | |
| Ethnic and racial identity | | |
| Socioeconomic status/ social class | | |
| Sexual orientation | | |
| Indigenous heritage | | |
| National origin | | |
| Gender | | |

(Based on ADDRESSING model; Hays, 2022)

**What do I struggle with about my own and others' diversity markers in society?**

Exercise 1.2

## SELF-REFLECTION ON BIASES AND INTERNALIZED STIGMAS

1. **Ask** yourself:
   a. What negative judgments have I noticed I make about others based on their race, gender, sexual orientation, religion, or any number of identity factors?

   b. What negative judgments have others made about my own identity characteristics? Which of these have I also had about myself or others who identify similarly?

   c. How do I feel about psychological therapy and how useful it would be for me personally if I were struggling with a mental health problem, or if someone in my family were struggling? Would I be embarrassed to receive therapy or have a close family member receive therapy?

2. **Try** an implicit association test that tries to assess your implicit, unconscious biases based on race, gender, stigma toward treatment, and so on. Doing such tests will allow you to access the quick negative judgements we might make about others based on identity factors, including biases and internalized stigma we may not even be aware that we have as mental health providers (Hall et al., 2015). Check out a range of such tests offered via Project Implicit: https://implicit.harv ard.edu/implicit/selectatest.html

   NOTE: This is simply to provide some additional information about your biases and should not be solely relied on as the only assessment of one's own biases.

3. **Engage** your peers and supervisors in an open, honest discussion about these observed internal biases or feelings of stigma toward therapy as a whole. A tip: Mention your own observations or struggles and encourage others to do the same so it feels less alienating or that the problem only lies in your own beliefs (most of us have biases, it's a part of human nature!). If you're a supervisor, share your own to encourage your trainees to do the same.

4. **Strategize** how you can overcome these biases, including being mindful of stigmatizing or negative thoughts during therapy with certain clients (or supervisors or supervisees), raising them in supervision or with close colleagues, or seeking your own therapy to better understand why these biases exist and how to address them so they do not impede the quality of care you provide.

Exercise 2.1

## Self-Reflection after a Therapeutic Rupture or Cultural Misstep Occurs

Consider the following questions to explore the therapeutic rupture, and use the spaces provided to **write your answers** for each to fully reflect on the situation.

1. Even before getting into the specifics of content of the misstep, explore: How do I know I made a possible cultural misstep or committed a microaggression? How did affect in the room change and what did that feel like? Was the client noticeably distressed/angry/sad/withdrawn, or was it subtler? Was it more about how I felt that cued me in to what happened?

    a. Ways I noticed that I made a misstep or performed a microaggression:

    \*\*\*\*\*\*\*\*\*\*\*\*\*\*\*\*\*\*\*\*\*\*\*\*\*\*\*\*\*\*\*\*\*\*\*\*\*\*\*\*\*\*\*\*\*\*\*\*\*\*\*\*\*\*\*\*\*\*\*\*\*\*\*\*\*\*

2. What were the sequences of events/interactions leading up to the noticeable shift in affect or visible emotional reaction from my client? That is, what was the exact nature/content of my misstep?

    a. Sequence of events leading to rupture:

    b. Content or nature of the cultural misstep:

    \*\*\*\*\*\*\*\*\*\*\*\*\*\*\*\*\*\*\*\*\*\*\*\*\*\*\*\*\*\*\*\*\*\*\*\*\*\*\*\*\*\*\*\*\*\*\*\*\*\*\*\*\*\*\*\*\*\*\*\*\*\*\*\*\*\*

3. What happened right after the rupture seems to have occurred, in terms of changes to the therapeutic alliance and session content? What is the likely impact of this rupture on future sessions and longer-term alliance with the client?

    a. Immediate consequences of the misstep/rupture:

    b. Possible long-term consequences of the misstep/rupture on therapeutic alliance/ability to meet therapeutic goals:

    \*\*\*\*\*\*\*\*\*\*\*\*\*\*\*\*\*\*\*\*\*\*\*\*\*\*\*\*\*\*\*\*\*\*\*\*\*\*\*\*\*\*\*\*\*\*\*\*\*\*\*\*\*\*\*\*\*\*\*\*\*\*\*\*\*\*

4. What are possible interpretations or internal reactions experienced by the client due to my misstep, based on (1) my understanding of their overall life experiences (e.g., other discriminatory experiences they have shared in session); (2) due to specific identity-related factors that they have expressed as salient/important to them; and (3) based on our own power-privilege differential in the therapist-client relationship?

   a. Possible interpretations/reactions by client:

   b. Client life experiences that may have contributed to their negative reaction to my misstep:

   c. Salient/important identity factors for client that were threatened by my misstep:

   d. Specific power or privilege differentials between my client and me that could enhance a negative reaction to my misstep:

   ***************************************************************

5. What did I feel internally as I committed the misstep, in terms of physical feelings and emotions? What thoughts were going through my head then? And how did I behaviorally react/what did I do if the misstep was immediately noticeable to me?

   a. Physical feelings when I realized I committed the misstep or I noticed a shift in alliance:

   b. Emotions:

   c. Thoughts:

   d. Behaviors:

Exercise 2.2

## REPAIRING CULTURAL MISSTEPS AND ACTIVELY PRACTICING CULTURAL HUMILITY

These are some ways to garner your sense of cultural humility and address cultural missteps or microaggressions you have committed towards others, which should be explored after thorough self-reflection as outlined in Exercise 2.1.

1. **Engage** your peers and supervisors in an open, honest discussion about your reflections about the misstep that occurred, in terms of what occurred, the client's reactions, your reactions, probable impacts on the therapeutic alliance, and possible threats to the therapeutic agenda. This includes sharing vulnerable feelings of internalized biases, your own societal messaging or life experiences underlying your committed misstep to better articulate and explicitly name your own cultural gaps in knowledge. A tip for supervisors/peers receiving this reflection: Share your own examples of missteps or relevant experiences that put you at risk for committing a microaggression, including your own power/privilege status with a trainee, to model this openness and crucial vulnerability in the cultural humility process.

2. **Strategize** with supervisors and peers about how you can raise the misstep directly and explicitly with the client in your next session, based on the client's own cultural background, interaction style, and specific symptoms that may intersect with such direct discussion. Explore how owning up to this mistake or explicitly addressing such a misstep with your client makes you feel, and how this fits into your own overall development as a therapist.

3. **Try** role-playing how you will raise and address the cultural misstep/microaggression with supervisors or colleagues prior to your session for practice. Think of adapting one of these statements:

   * *X, before we get started with our session agenda for today, I just wanted to raise something that happened last week that has been on my mind. Specifically, I want to apologize for when I said/did XYZ last week, and I am sorry if that was hurtful to you.*
   * *As your therapist, I always strive to provide the most open, accepting, and safe environment for you to reach your goals, and by doing XYZ [be explicit, no excuses!], I violated that promise of such a safe space. That is not in line with my professional values, and I am truly sorry that I behaved in such a way. I felt [shame, guilt, anger at myself, sadness] by how I behaved/what I said.*

* *Would you be open to sharing how you felt or what you thought when I said/did XYZ? What was that like for you?*
* *How can I rebuild your trust or help you feel comfortable and accepted/ safe in session moving forward? I think we have already had a lot of positive progress towards your goals of ABC, and I want to do whatever I can to make sure my mistake does not move us away from continuing to achieve your goals.* [Be ready with a few ways you can suggest on your own, if your client isn't sure, so it doesn't fall all on them].

4. **Be brave and address your misstep** with your client by doing what you practiced with others. This is your final step of learning cultural humility, and trust me—it gets easier and becomes more second-nature with repeated practice!

Exercise 4.1

DETERMINING WHETHER AND HOW TO ENGAGE IN SELF-EDUCATION ABOUT
SPECIFIC CULTURAL NORMS THAT MAY BE INFLUENCING THE PRESENTING
PROBLEM WITH A CLIENT

After self-reflection on your knowledge and familiarity with the identity facets for your specific case in mind, start with the main stem question 1 below, and then review the recommendations for specific educational or scientific resources to use accordingly:

1. Are there salient parts of my client's identity that I definitely know are related to the presenting problems or treatment targets (either through assessment and/or explicit discussion with my client)? **If no, go to step 2. If yes, skip to steps 3–5. If you're unsure, review Chapter 3** on assessing for this more directly with your client, and then ask yourself this question again.

2. Even if upon assessment of identity-related factors you have a client who is not endorsing a connection of these factors to their target symptoms, it is not a bad idea to at least engage in **some initial review of major cultural rules/norms** for the identity factor you guess to be most relevant to the presenting concerns (using your clinical intuition and conceptualization skills, ideally with some consultation/supervision). In this case, a review of the literature is at least warranted (look at the following **recommendation 3**, and only progress to subsequent steps if the identity factor becomes more saliently related to your therapeutic work or is revealed in repeated assessment to be connected to your therapeutic goals).

3. A first step across scenarios is **reviewing the empirical or published practice literature** on (ideally) the overlap between the specific cultural (and intersectional) identities of your client and how these have been studied in the specific disorder at hand, or if too narrow, then how these identities have been studied within the context of psychopathology/clinical psychology more broadly. Such a review will provide insight into the pooled knowledge (if any exists) for the clients we are working with, so we are not starting from scratch.

4. Next, **work with your client to identify someone** they ideally trust (and know personally, or can endorse as being a cultural authority in their current, local context) to be a representative of their particular cultural identity, i.e., a steward with whom you and the client would be comfortable talking to together (or you individually, if the client prefers) about how specific cultural norms overlay with the client's chief mental health symptoms. This individual will also be able to provide the therapist with important instruction on specific cultural practices, beliefs, or challenges, so this burden does not fall on the client to "teach" the therapist about their identity factors. Further, such consultation with a cultural steward may provide better understanding

about intersectional identity challenges your client may be facing, and will ideally provide better situational context about how your client's identities interact with the immediate societal environment.

5. **Share** with colleagues and supervisors about what you have learned in terms of the cultural norms and nuances at hand from both published and cultural steward sources to **obtain additional consultation and guidance** around whether your conceptualization about how these cultural norms overlay with treatment targets (and the treatment itself) is accurate, or whether you are still grappling with any crucial gaps in knowledge. Ask for suggestions for how such cultural values will need to be incorporated in your treatment plan (if applicable), particularly from colleagues and supervisors who have expertise in that specific cultural/identity group or have had their own extensive experience working with specific diverse populations.

Exercise 6.1

ADDRESSING MICROAGGRESSIONS WHEN WE OBSERVE OTHERS IN OUR
PROFESSIONAL SETTINGS COMMITTING THEM TOWARD OUR CLIENTS

**1. Reflect here on what specifically happened that you believe was a microaggression directed toward your or another's client.**

What specifically happened? What was the microinsult/microassault that occurred, and who was the target and the perpetrator?

Nature of microaggression: _____

Perpetrator (identity, role, etc.):_____

Target (identity, role, etc.):_____

**2. When this incident occurred, what did you feel? What thoughts came up, and did you have an immediate or delayed recognition that a microaggression had occurred?**

_____

_____

**3. When this incident occurred, how did others (if applicable) react or respond?**

_____

_____

**4. What can you say to practice naming the specific microaggression that occurred explicitly?**

_____

_____

_____

* If you didn't say this when it occurred, and you're reflecting on this after the incident has already occurred, when can you next state what you came up with above with the offending individual?

_____

**5. What language can you use that is appropriate within that setting (whether it's within a clinical team meeting versus a group treatment session and your target is a colleague versus another client) to express your clear disapproval of the microaggression to disarm it?**

_____

_____

_____

**6. What kind of education might be most effective to provide to the offender to explain why their words or actions were microaggressive? List a few points you could refer to here.**

Point 1: _____

Point 2: _____

Point 3: _____

**7. Who can you approach in your clinical team, organization, or administration to share what happened and obtain more institutional/broader support around this incident to ensure it is addressed more fully by your practice setting?**

Colleagues: _____

Supervisors: _____

Administrators: _____

External scholars/Networks: _____

_____

Exercise 7.1

CHECKLIST WORKSHEET FOR INCORPORATING IDENTIFIED IDENTITY-RELATED STRENGTHS AND RESOURCES INTO TREATMENT

Did I (check each one as you complete, ideally chronologically):

☐ **Assess for identity-related strengths/resources that may be incorporated into treatment?**

Which ones, specifically?

  ☐ Culture-specific skills and knowledge (e.g., community naturalistic/medicinal health expertise, cooking, storytelling)

  ☐ Culture-specific coping strategies (e.g., cultural metaphors for understanding emotional symptoms, interpersonal activities that are culturally relevant or valued)

  ☐ Specific community resources (e.g., identity-related political or social causes, places for worship, or financial resources)

  ☐ Artistic outlets for processing of emotional material (e.g., culture-specific dance, art, and music)

☐ **Work with peers/supervisors and do my own assessment of which specific parts of my current EST protocol would be most appropriate to incorporate identified strengths?**

☐ **Broach the topic and explain the rationale to client so they are empowered and informed about my intention to bring such identity-related strengths into our work together?**

**Have I continued to check in with client about using such specific identity-related strengths, resources, or activities after our initial conversation?**

  ☐ Yes, I have brought up the topic again after the first time.

  ☐ No, I have not revisited the topic.

If not, why haven't I done so? _____

_____

Do I need to reconsider bringing it up again? When might it be helpful to consider doing so?

_____

_____

_____

Exercise 8.1

CHECKLIST OF GUIDELINES FOR RELAPSE-PREVENTION TREATMENT PLANNING

Use this list to jot down which guidelines may be relevant and what points specific to your client you might want to raise for each. For guidelines that are not relevant or not high priority to touch on, simply indicate N/A, but a general rule of thumb is that 2–3 guidelines are likely highly applicable to your client.

**Guideline 1: Exploring Your Own Cultural Identity, Beliefs, and Biases Before Providing Therapy**

_____

_____

_____

**Guideline 2: Practicing Cultural Humility as a Continuous Process**

_____

_____

_____

**Guideline 3: Balancing Culturally Informed and Individualized Assessment of the Presenting Problem**

_____

_____

_____

**Guideline 4: Engaging in Self-Education about Specific Cultural Norms Using a Variety of Sources**

_____

_____

_____

**Guideline 5: Addressing Stigma and Other Cultural Barriers to Psychological Treatment**

_____

_____

_____

**Guideline 6: Exploring the Impact of Discrimination and Microaggressions on Therapy**

_____

_____

_____

**Guideline 7: Identifying and Incorporating Cultural Strengths and Resources into Treatment**

_____

_____

_____

Exercise 9.1

## SUPERVISOR REFLECTION OF POWER, PRIVILEGE, AND BIASES TOWARD SUPERVISEES

Think about the following questions as they relate specifically to your supervisee. Answer as honestly and openly as you can, to fully understand which aspects might potentially facilitate or hinder the ideal working relationship in clinical supervision.

1. **Reflection on identity and power/privilege differentials between you and your supervisee:**

a. What are some of the salient identity differences and similarities you believe you share with your supervisee? Think broadly about identity on multiple facets of one's identity (e.g., anchoring back to the ADDRESSING model by Hays, 2022).

**Differences in identity:** _____

**Similarities in identity:** _____

b. How about in terms of the power and privilege you hold as a supervisor? How does this further intersect with these identity differences and/or similarities?

i. **Nature of the power differential between me and my supervisee:**

_____

**This could impact our working relationship in the following ways:**

_____

ii. **Nature of the privilege differential between me and my supervisee:**

_____

**This could impact our working relationship in the following ways:**

_____

2. **Reflection on your own biases as a supervisor or specifically in terms of salient identity markers for your supervisee:**

a. What negative judgments have I noticed I make about my supervisees based on a range of factors (their level of training, type of training, or a host of identity markers such as race, gender, sexual orientation, religion, etc.)?

_____

_____

b. Have I noticed that any of these negative thoughts/judgments come up in the context of working with this particular supervisee?

_____

_____

c. Being honest with myself, have I observed that these negative beliefs have impacted the way I have treated my supervisee or how I have engaged with them in the context of clinical supervision? Be specific here about what these behaviors have been.

_____

_____

d. Having written down the ways I may have behaved in biased ways with my trainee, how do I feel about it? How is this behavior in line or in contrast with my core values as a supervisor?

_____

_____

_____

Chapter Boxes and Tables

*Table 2.1* COMMON CULTURAL MISSTEPS

| Microaggressions | Case Conceptualization | Interaction Style |
|---|---|---|
| Maltreatment of clients directly based on their identity (race/ethnicity, culture, gender, sexual orientation, disability status etc.) | Conflating one's own value systems/beliefs/biases with clinical conceptualization of maintaining symptoms and subsequent goals for treatment | Unintentionally interacting in ways with clients that emphasize their difference in identity from you or the "mainstream" culture, effectively "othering" the client over repeated interactions |
| • Verbal insults (e.g., using offensive or incorrect terms, mispronunciation of names)<br>• Nonverbal discriminatory behaviors (e.g., guarded body language, disapproving facial expressions)<br>• Use of stereotypical tropes when describing clients in context of clinical supervision or clinical reports (e.g., "as is typical for African people . . .") | • Superimposing our own values about ideal family systems and interpersonal dynamics in therapy targets for clients (e.g., how close children should be to their parents or should move out of their family home, what romantic relationships should look like)<br>• Incorporating our own beliefs in treatment targets when not raised by client (e.g., pushing clients to espouse feminist values, encouraging clients to solely align with individualistic values)<br>• Assuming that a client completely adheres to their cultural or identity background practices or only to their individually-valued practices, instead of a combination of both | • Comments about the client's own communication (e.g., repeatedly noting difficulties in understanding their accent, or asking about where they are from if they don't readily share)<br>• Use of categorizing terms that actively separate them from us as the therapists (e.g., "your community," "where you come from," instead of directly naming their community such as "being Arab American")<br>• Specifically avoiding engaging in any appropriate levels of self-disclosure about your own identity/background, thereby solidifying a power/privilege boundary, particularly where these concepts are already quite salient |

*Table 3.1* SAMPLE STANDARDIZED ASSESSMENT MEASURES

| Self-Report Measures | Semi-Structured Interviews |
|---|---|
| **Discrimination measures:**<br>Everyday Discrimination Scale (EDS)<br>　　(Williams et al., 1997)<br><br>Detroit Area Study Discrimination<br>Questionnaire<br>　　(Jackson & Williams, 2002) | **UConn Racial/Ethnic Stress and**<br>**Trauma Survey (UnRESTS)**<br>　　(Williams, Metzger,<br>　　　Leins, & DeLapp, 2018)<br><br>* Specifically incorporates assessment<br>　of discrimination and racial trauma,<br>　using the CFI (see next) as the<br>　foundation |
| **Acculturative Stress:**<br>Multidimensional Acculturative Stress<br>Inventory (MASI)<br>　　(Rodriguez, Myers, Mira, Flores, &<br>Garcia-Hernandez, 2002)<br><br>Vancouver Acculturation Index (VIA)<br>　　(Ryder, Alden, & Paulhus, 2000) | ----------<br><br>**DSM-5 Cultural Formulation**<br>**Interview (CFI)**<br>　　(American Psychiatric<br>　　Association, 2013) |
| **Cultural Values/Orientation:**<br>Singelis Self-Construal scale (SCS)<br>　　(Singelis, 1994)<br><br>Culture Orientation Scale<br>　　(Triandis & Gelfland, 1998) | * Provides a cultural formulation<br>　integrated with DSM-5 diagnosis,<br>　found in appendix of DSM-5 |
| **Ethnic Identity:**<br>Multigroup Ethnic Identity Measure (MEIM)<br>　　(Roberts et al., 1999)<br><br>Ethnic Identity Scale (EIS)<br>　　(Umaña-Taylor, Yazedjian, &<br>　　Bámaca-Gómez, 2004) | ----------<br><br>**Brief Cultural Interview (BCI)**<br><br>　　(Groen, Richters, Laban, &<br>　　Devillé, 2017) |
| **Stigma toward mental health treatment:**<br>Self-Stigma of Seeking Help (SSOSH)<br>　　(Vogel, Wade, & Haake, 2006)<br><br>Stigma-9 Questionnaire (STIG-9)<br>　　(Gierk, Löwe, Murray, & Kohlmann, 2018) | * Primarily tested in immigrant/<br>　refugee populations in the<br>　Netherlands, at a more preliminary<br>　stage but shows promise given its<br>　brevity |

Box 3.1

This is by no means an exhaustive list, but it will hopefully get you started on thinking about how to raise identity-related influences within your assessment of the presenting problem. These prompts can also be posed to clients for continuous case conceptualization at various points over the course of therapy, not just at the beginning of treatment.

Note: If you're using a semi-structured standardized assessment/diagnostic interview, you can also add the following questions to round out your assessment and ensure you are examining the influence of identity factors within this more structured context. Depending on your practice policies, you just may not be able to ask as many follow-up questions and may be required to leave this for the first therapy sessions. Regardless, it's important to at least mention the first stem to open up the space for the client to discuss these issues.

* [FOLLOWING PSYCHOSOCIAL HISTORY AND EVALUATION OF CHIEF COMPLAINT]. *Thank you for providing information on why you are seeking services and telling me a little bit about your life outside of your most troubling symptoms. One last thing I wanted to raise was that you mentioned that* [XYZ identity factor] *is important to you* [OR] *that you identify as* [XYZ identity factor], *and I just wanted to understand whether you think that being* [XYZ identity factor] *influences the main symptoms of* [specific disorder] *we talked about today? This could be both in terms of how these identities make your symptoms worse, but also if you think they help you cope with your symptoms better.*

* [FOLLOW-UP TO THIS PREVIOUS QUESTION IF CLIENT IS UNSURE WHAT YOU MEAN]: *So, what I mean is that often individuals coming into our clinic will mention that they identify with a particular race, religion, gender, or even specific community. Since we are more than our mental health symptoms, we like to know about how our clients identify in these other ways so we can understand you as a person more fully. Also, sometimes those very identities (or a combination of them) can impact the mental health symptoms we are trying to help you target in therapy, either in positive ways (like giving you a healthy way to cope with feeling depressed or lonely, for example) or in negative ways (like feeling down about how your symptoms affect your community or are not in line with your community's values), or even a combination. Do you think your identity influences anything we have spoken about so far today? It is totally fine if it does not, but I just want to make sure I do not miss something important that might be part of what is going on for you or that may help us come up with the most useful treatment plan.*

* [IF CLIENT ENDORSES INFLUENCE OF IDENTITY FACTOR(S) ON CURRENT TREATMENT-SEEKING, ASK THEM TO TELL YOU AS MUCH AS THEY ARE COMFORTABLE DOING AND THEN]: *Thank you so much for sharing that insight on how being* [XYZ identity factor, explicitly stated, avoid using generalities] *might have an influence on the symptoms that brought you into the assessment today. We will likely come back to this discussion throughout the therapy periodically to continue to explore how these identity factors continue to play a role. But you can also feel free to bring these up any time over the course of your treatment with us, this is always a welcome space to do so.*
* [IF CLIENT DENIES ANY INFLUENCE/RELEVANCE OF IDENTITY FACTORS]: *That's completely fine if you do not think how you identify* [or being XYZ] *has a significant impact on what we have discussed so far in terms of your mental health symptoms. If that changes, and you want to raise the discussion again in the future over the course of your treatment with us, I just want you to know that there is always a welcome space to do so here.*
* [FOLLOW-UP CHECK-IN AT FUTURE SESSIONS ABOUT INFLUENCE OF IDENTITY FACTORS]: *If you might recall, when we first were trying to figure out your main symptoms and what we wanted to target in the beginning of treatment, we discussed how being* [XYZ identity factor] *might be related to what we're targeting in treatment, in either helpful or unhelpful ways. I remember that at that time, we discussed that your symptoms were impacted in terms of* [FILL IN FROM PREVIOUS DISCUSSIONS] [OR] *did not feel impacted by these identities at the time. I'm curious whether this feels any different right now, and if so, how? What do you think the impact of being* [XYZ identity factor] *is on your symptoms at the current time?*

*Table 4.1* LOCAL AND REGIONAL CULTURAL CONSULTATION RESOURCES

| Local | National/Regional | Networks/Repositories |
|---|---|---|
| Check website (or telephone) listings for locally based: | Look for mental health organizations specifically catering to the needs of distinct identity groups, such as:[1,2] | Check out written resources pooled together by clinicians and researchers working with a variety of diverse communities, such as:[1,2] |
| * Religious institutions<br>* Community social service or employment/ immigration agencies<br>* Cultural organizations (e.g., those putting together cultural events/fairs)<br>* State-level or city-level health disparities offices or community outreach teams<br>* Community mental health clinics located in neighborhoods with diverse clientele<br>* Language centers where various languages are taught | * National Alliance for Hispanic Health<br>* Indian Health Service (INS)<br>* Human Rights Campaign (HRC)<br>* National Deaf Center (NDC)<br>* Rural Health Information Hub | * Mental Health America (MHA) community-specific programs<br>* National Alliance for Mental Illness (NAMI), which has various community-specific pages/repositories<br>* Substance Abuse and Mental Health Services Administration (SAMHSA) Faith-Based and Community Initiatives |

Notes:

[1]This is NOT an exhaustive list! Find similar resources for any other specific identity group you wish to learn more about and rely on registered/recommended organizations versus individual/ unverified resources online.

[2]Weblinks for these listed organizations are at the end of this book in the Appendix under "Resources".

Box 5.1

Sample Prompts to Explore and Address Potential Cultural Barriers to Therapy Engagement

We explore some sample prompts to examine potential impact of the major cultural barriers discussed in this chapter; obviously, there may be other cultural barriers at play not covered here, and these prompts hopefully provide some model for how to address other barriers you detect as well.

## Stigma toward Mental Health and/or Treatment

* **Normalizing stigma towards mental health/treatment:** *I work with a number of clients who have shared with me that sometimes their friends, family members, or communities at large have some negative beliefs about mental health or going to therapy. Is that true for you? I would love to hear what some of those beliefs are so I can understand what that may look like in your unique case.*
* **Using appropriate self-disclosure:** *You know, I grew up in a household where mental health wasn't that valued or often not well understood. It took a lot of work for me to even try to understand why it might be important, and to do the work I do now. I wonder if you have experienced anything similar to me?*
* **Setting up the stage to gently challenge stigmatizing beliefs:** *You have spoken positively about how much your identity as someone from a rural Midwestern town means to you, and I know how important this part of your background is to you. What are some beliefs you hold in high regard or have positively influenced who you are today that you feel are connected to your upbringing in a rural, closely knit, small town?* [AFTER DISCUSSION]: *Have there been beliefs from this same part of your identity that you think are not the most helpful or important to you?* [AFTER DISCUSSION, IF MENTAL HEALTH BELIEFS DON'T ORGANICALLY ARISE]: *I'm curious, are any of the beliefs that have positively impacted you or that you don't see as relevant to what you value about yourself related to how you feel about mental health or even coming to therapy?* [GIVE SPACE TO DISCUSS WITHOUT FEELING YOU NEED TO DIRECTLY CHALLENGE AT FIRST].

## DISCREPANCIES IN EXPECTATIONS FOR IDEAL THERAPEUTIC RELATIONSHIP

* **More directive line of questioning:** *XXX, before we continue on our agenda for today, I wanted to ask you about how therapy is going.*

*Specifically, how do you feel about how you and I are working together? Have you found my style of presenting information or leading us through the treatment skills to be helpful or unhelpful? Is there anything I can do that would be more in line with what you were hoping I would be like when you were looking for a therapist?* [AFTER DISCUSSION]: *Thank you so much for sharing how you were kind of envisioning it, and those expectations make a lot of sense based on what we have discussed about your background in terms of* [BE SPECIFIC HERE IF YOU KNOW]. *I want to share a bit about how I think about therapy* [AS A PARTNERSHIP, A COACH, WHATEVER YOUR ORIENTATION IS].

* **Less directive line of questioning:** *XXX, before we continue on our agenda for today, I wanted to ask you a bit about what you think about therapy generally. What do you think a therapist is supposed to be like, and before you came here, what did you think therapy was going to look like?*

* **Gently raising how a discrepancy may be impacting therapy:** *So now that we have both shared what we think the ideal therapy relationship looks like, it seems like there are certainly some differences. I think it's very fair to think of a therapist as being someone who* [FILL IN SPECIFICS FROM WHAT CLIENT SHARED HERE], *and I get that looks different from my training to approach therapy as the therapist who* [FILL IN SPECIFICS FROM YOUR ORIENTATION HERE TO HIGHLIGHT ANY DISCREPANCY]. *I think one thing we both see similarly, however, is that we both want you to get the most out of therapy by* [STATE THERAPEUTIC GOALS WHETHER SYMPTOM REDUCTION OR IMPROVEMENT IN FUNCTIONING, ETC]. *To be able to achieve that shared goal, I wonder if we can find a way to reconcile or find a middle ground between the different ways you prefer a therapist to be and the way I am most used to providing care. Are you open to us coming up with a few ideas of how to find a compromise so we can help you get the most out of therapy?*

## Mistrust/Hesitation Working with a Therapist from a Different Identity Background

* **Open-ended exploration of potential mistrust/hesitation:** *XXX, before we continue on our agenda for today, I wanted to ask you about how therapy is going. Specifically, how comfortable are you feeling about working with me specifically as your therapist? I know it's never easy to talk about difficult things, but is there anything I can do to make you feel more comfortable or most safe to share what's going on for you?*

* **Taking ownership/using self-disclosure:** *I just wanted to make sure I asked this because I am very aware that I am* [NAME SALIENT POWER/PRIVILEGE DIFFERENTIAL OR IDENTITY DIFFERENCE], *and that can make the therapy relationship already tricky, because it*

*requires you to be more vulnerable with me. I am so appreciative for everything you share with me, and don't take anything you show the courage to share with me for granted or lightly. I know first-hand that when you feel really different or vulnerable with someone else that it can be difficult to share everything going on. For instance, as a female in a primarily male-dominated science field, I often am concerned about being mistreated or that my opinions may be swept aside in professional settings where there are mostly men* [OR NAME ANY OF YOUR OWN AUTHENTIC POWER/PRIVILEGE/IDENTITY FACETS/RELEVANT SITUATIONS]. *Do you ever feel similarly hesitant to share anything with me either because I am your therapist, a woman, White, or grew up in the United States, or really, anything else about my identity?* [BE SPECIFIC HERE ABOUT HOW YOU DIFFER ACROSS INTERSECTIONAL FACETS, NOT ASSUMING ONE AREA OF DIFFERENCE].

* **Showing commitment to the therapeutic alliance:** *I want to make sure I do whatever I can to ensure that you get the most out of therapy, because I know it takes away your time and money to come here. I am committed to doing whatever I need to do as your therapist to make this a safe and open place where, even if we are different from each other in a number of ways or a few very important ones, you feel comfortable in sharing what you want to so you can get the most out of our work together.*

* **Modeling how to brainstorm ways to address the mistrust:** *I think it's very reasonable to be hesitant with me because I'm* [BE SPECIFIC HERE IF CLIENT PROVIDES THIS INFORMATION; DON'T ASSUME], *thank you so much for sharing that. I have a few ideas of how I can show you that you can trust me and hopefully this may help you feel more comfortable working with me, even if it takes some time, that's okay. For instance, we can make more space in our sessions for you to share anything you want to about how you have experienced other instances of discrimination based on your* [STATE SPECIFIC IDENTITY FACTOR HERE] *so we can better explore where this reasonable hesitation of yours comes from. I can also regularly check in about how I might be myself perpetuating some of this mistreatment based on your* [IDENTITY FACTOR], *to make sure I can check myself and immediately address anything I'm doing to make you feel hesitant about how much you can trust me. I am also happy to share some of my own experiences with how I have learned to build trust in vulnerable situations so you don't feel alone with having to do so. Another thing I am happy to do is to see if I have another client from a similar background who is willing to talk with you about how they felt working with me (without me being privy to that conversation) so you can get a more unbiased idea of whether I am a good fit for what you need, only if you and they are both comfortable doing so, of course. Do any of these feel like they may be helpful?*

*Table 6.1* WHAT TO DO WHEN YOUR CLIENT RAISES EXPERIENCES OF PREVIOUS DISCRIMINATION IN THERAPY

| **Validate and empathize** with their experience | In the initial report, **let the client lead** the level of detail and feelings they want to share about their experience | **Express a commitment** to doing your best to ensure you don't discriminate or perform microaggressions as a therapist |
|---|---|---|
| <u>Try</u>: "I'm so sorry you had to experience that. That must have been so difficult, and I am so glad you brought it up here." | <u>Try</u>: "I'm here to listen to anything you want to share about that experience, in terms of what happened and/or what you felt. There is no pressure to share more than you feel comfortable doing." | <u>Try</u>: "I definitely want this to be a place where you feel safe, not judged and one where you feel completely valued for who you are. I will work hard to make sure I do everything I need to for our therapy to be that place for you. I will always be open to hearing if you ever feel like it's not so I can correct what I need to in my behavior to make sure it is." |
| <u>AVOID</u>: "Are you sure that really is what that person meant? Could it be that they didn't mean anything discriminatory?" | <u>AVOID</u>: "Can you tell me exactly what was said or what happened next? Tell me more about how that made you feel and let's break down what happened for everyone involved." | <u>AVOID</u>: "Please make sure you explain to me or tell me when I might be committing a microaggression. I won't be able to tell I'm doing so or address the situation unless you let me know, so please make sure you do." |

Box 6.2

## How Can I Be Mindful about NOT Committing Microaggressions in Therapy?

* *Engage in self-reflection about your own current biases as we cover in Guideline 1 (remember: this is continuous process throughout your career!).*

* *Discuss these potential areas of judgment/bias with supervisors and peers to generate ways for you to address them outside of your time with your client.*

* *During sessions with clients, notice your negative reactions and thoughts to their salient identity markers; if in-the-moment awareness is difficult for you, reflect and write about how you felt in the session or watch videos/listen to sessions to see if you can more objectively view your body language/verbal expressions that may be related to your own biases.*

* *If there are still gaps in our knowledge about where our own biases may lie, consider engaging in implicit bias tests or other exercises that help us tap into such biases that may be at play outside of conscious awareness (see end of Chapter 6 and text resources for more on this).*

Box 7.1

Consider the following questions that you may pose to clients to more explicitly raise the possibility of incorporating culturally relevant strengths across some different types of ESTs (note: this is a subsample, not an exhaustive list of ESTs, and you're encouraged to think about how these can be modified for other treatment approaches):

*   **Broad prompts to explore:** *What would you say are your strengths, talents, or abilities that people in your family, community, or social network recognize, value, or appreciate about you? What do others in your life say you're good at? What do you believe you bring to relationships with others that you see as a positive part of who you are or what you're capable of? This can be in terms of certain skills you are known to be good at/you feel that you're good at, personality characteristics you are valued for in your family/community, or certain knowledge that you can contribute to certain situations that maybe others don't have as much of.* [THEN THIS INFORMATION CAN BE USED FOR ANY OF THE MORE EST-SPECIFIC PROMPTS BELOW.]
*   **For behavioral activation approaches:** *As we think about ways to help increase your daily pleasure and motivation, it sometimes helps to include activities that are personally relevant for us so we feel more genuinely motivated to do them. For instance, I have had clients mention that certain cultural practices, political or social activism, religious involvement, or specific family activities, just to name a few examples, are some things that they used to feel a lot of joy about doing before they got depressed. Are there any activities that are maybe connected to specific parts of your life or identities that we should consider adding into your weekly activity scheduling?*
*   **For exposure therapy approaches**: *It's sometimes helpful for us to put items on our exposure hierarchies that allow us to face our fears to do something that is personally relevant to us or tied to a bigger part of ourselves, like maybe a community we belong to, something particularly important to our families, or something that is connected to or affirms a part of our identity. Can you think of any things you're avoiding that are particularly upsetting because they are otherwise really important to you and that you would do if you didn't feel anxious?*
*   **For cognitive therapy approaches:** *You have mentioned that your family/ community is pretty aware that you often have depressive/suicidal/anxious thoughts. What are some ways that your loved ones have helped you gently challenge those thoughts in a way that doesn't feel judgmental but instead, supportive? I often observe that there are some nuggets of wisdom in the ways our communities/families try to support us when we have difficult*

*thoughts, and I'd love to explore if we could use any of those helpful approaches as we practice cognitive restructuring/challenging in our work together.*

* **For mindfulness and values-based approaches:** *As we explore the values that are most personally relevant to us and that we want to live our lives by, it is undeniable that our identities, whether it's our particular cultural background, gender, religion, age, sexual orientation or any number of identity factors that make us who we are, can influence what values are most important to us. While I want to encourage you to think about what values are most important to you (and not just your family/community), I completely get that for many of us, our values are greatly connected to those specific parts of our identities that are most important to us. I'd love for this to be a space where we can talk about what you have noticed about some of your own strengths in your family and community systems, and how these might be connected to how you want to be in the world and the values that are most important to you. What might some of those strengths that you value in your relationships within your community or shared community values be that you hold in high regard?* [IDEALLY EXPLICITLY NAME THE IDENTITY FACET(S) THAT THE CLIENT HAS ALREADY RAISED AS MOST SALIENT INSTEAD OF USING SUCH GENERAL TERMS HERE.]

* **For relapse prevention phases of treatment:** *In order to maintain all the progress you have made in therapy, it's helpful for us to keep thinking about how you can practice what you have learned here in areas that are personally relevant to you, even long after therapy is done.* [RETURN TO FIRST BROAD PROMPT, AND DISCUSS APPLICATION OF IDENTIFIED STRENGTHS/RESOURCES CONNECTED TO IDENTITY FACETS IN THE SHORT, MEDIUM, AND LONG TERM.]

Box 9.1

SAMPLE PROMPTS TO ADDRESS INSTANCES WHERE YOU HAVE COMMITTED A MICROAGGRESSION TOWARD YOUR SUPERVISEE WITHIN THE CONTEXT OF SUPERVISION

If you are aware that you have committed a microaggression toward your supervisee, well done. This is half the battle, and now it's time to fix the misstep and to try to preserve the clinical supervision relationship. Remember your core values, and be brave to accept fault, regardless of the power differential that exists. And as always, this list gives you some ideas of how to raise the issue, but certainly consult with colleagues where you can, to get additional support, guidance, and ideas. Remember, by raising your own missteps with supervisees, you are modeling cultural humility for their own training, while simultaneously engaging in an act of social justice to reduce the disparities and disproportionately poorer treatment faced by supervisees from underrepresented backgrounds.

Sample prompts to bring this up in your supervision meeting or to explore whether such microaggressions have occurred without your awareness:

* *X, before we get started with reviewing your clients today, I just wanted to raise something that happened last week that has been on my mind. Specifically, I want to apologize for when I said/did XYZ* [**be explicit about what it was! Don't be vague**] *last week, and I am sorry if that was hurtful to you. I have been doing my own reflection about my values as a supervisor, and I realize that I have some of my own biases or preconceived notions about clinical supervision that might have clouded the way I treated you. This is not fair to you, and I am truly sorry for that.*

* *As your clinical supervisor, I am here to support you and provide the best training I can to you. It is my intention to always strive to provide the most open, accepting, and safe environment for you to reach your training goals, and by doing XYZ* [**be explicit, no excuses!**]*, I violated that promise of such a safe space. That is not in line with my professional values, and I am truly sorry that I behaved in such a way. I felt* [**shame, guilt, anger at myself, sadness, etc.**] *by how I behaved/what I said.*

* *Would you be open to sharing how you felt or what you thought when I said/did XYZ? What was that like for you?*

* *I am working hard on my own self-reflection about when I commit behaviors that are unacceptable or unfair to you, but I would love to create a space where you feel comfortable letting me know when I inadvertently act in similar ways or am offensive to you. What are some ways I can make you feel like this is a professional relationship where you can raise those types of concerns?*

* Are there any other instances of mistreatment or biased behavior from your perspective that we haven't talked about that you are comfortable bringing up right now? It's totally okay if there isn't, I know I have some work to do to make you trust that this is a safe space to discuss such issues within our supervision relationship. But if you have anything to raise while we are discussing it today, I'm all ears.

Box 9.2

It can be really hard to raise issues of mistreatment when you're on the receiving end of it, and particularly with someone who inherently holds power over your training and part of your professional trajectory. While we all hope that supervisors will themselves raise the issues, some are unwilling but many are also unaware that they have engaged in behavior that is biased or microaggressive. Don't automatically assume a negative intention by your supervisor; check your own experiences that may be categorizing your supervisor as someone else who has been intentionally discriminatory, and see if you can approach the situation with an openness and with compassion. And what if after attempting to address the issue with your supervisor, it doesn't work? Well, then it's time to get the support you deserve elsewhere, as outlined after these sample prompts for first trying to raise the issue directly with your supervisor.

Sample prompts to bring up an instance of biased behavior by your supervisor or general feelings of being dismissed or unfairly treated (ideally in an individual meeting with your supervisor to reduce defensiveness by your supervisor, if this feels safe to do so):

* *X, before we get started with reviewing my clients today, I just wanted to raise something that happened last week that has been on my mind. Specifically, I wanted to share that when you said/did XYZ* [**be as explicit as you can so there is no confusion about what occurred**] *last week, I felt* [**anger, sadness, disappointment, surprise, etc.**] *because this felt like unfair treatment* **OR** *that I was being singled out based on my XX identity* **OR** *it didn't take my XX identity facet into account, and that felt disrespectful/disappointing. Can we spend some of our supervision time today talking about that some more?*
* *I want to get the most out of supervision with you, and while our focus is on providing the best clinical care to my clients that you supervise, when these types of interactions occur between you and me, it makes me feel less able to do that or engage in our clinical supervision to my full capacity. I would like to talk about how we can discuss differences between us in terms of our backgrounds or perspectives about therapy so that we can be respectful of each other's perspectives and get the most out of supervision. Would this be possible to spend some time doing this? It's important to me.*
* [**If this feels safe and authentic to do**] *I have faced a lot of discrimination over my lifetime in other personal and professional contexts, particularly directed towards* [**name specific or intersectional identity facets here**], *and it has been a challenge for me to experience similar dynamics here. I want to be able to have a supervision relationship where we can discuss*

*these issues and I can raise these experiences if they occur in supervision*
*with you without a fear of being dismissed or those experiences being*
*minimized. I would value having such an open dialogue with you and*
*I think it would be great for both our professional relationship and in terms*
*of my broader training.*

In sum, you can raise your own feelings about what specific instances or features of your interaction with your supervisor feel discriminatory or biased, while still stating an intention to build a strong working alliance and training relationship with them.

But what if they are not responsive, become defensive, or dismiss your concerns as unimportant? If you have given it a try to raise this directly with your supervisor, here are some others you can go to, depending on your comfort level and specific interpersonal/department/training clinic dynamics. Note, each will have different levels of support they can provide, from informal suggestions or guidance of what to do next, to disciplinary ability. A good rule of thumb is to start with someone who can provide more support and a listening ear about best next steps, who may provide a few more suggestions of how to address the issue again with your supervisor, or who may alternatively advise you to immediately "dial up" your report of this behavior, because of a standing pattern of mistreatment or due to the egregiousness of it. That next level of outreach typically can help you come to a more formal resolution or administrative-level intervention.

INITIAL

- * Senior trainee/colleague
- * Another faculty member in your training area
- * External colleagues/scholars/mentors (not at your training setting or institution)

NEXT STEPS

- * Another supervisor on your team
- * Director of clinical training/clinic director

Resources and Further Reading

## Key Texts and Guidelines for Overall Multicultural Practice

American Psychological Association. (2017). Multicultural guidelines: An ecological approach to context, identity and intersectionality. http://www.apa.org/about/policy/multicultural-guidelines.pdf

Asnaani, A., Majeed, I. M., Kaur, K., & Gutierrez Chavez, M. (2022). Diversity and clinical perspectives in psychology. In G. Asmundson (Ed.), *Comprehensive clinical psychology* (2nd ed., pp. 202–224). Elsevier. https://doi.org/10.1016/B978-0-12-818697-8.00081-9

Bernal, G., Jiménez-Chafey, M. I., & Domenech Rodríguez, M. M. (2009). Cultural adaptation of treatments: A resource for considering culture in evidence-based practice. *Professional Psychology: Research and Practice, 40*(4), 361–368. https://doi.org/10.1037/a0016401

Cross, T. (2003). Culture as a resource for mental health. *Cultural Diversity and Ethnic Minority Psychology, 9,* 354–359.

Danso, R. (2018). Cultural competence and cultural humility: A critical reflection on key cultural diversity concepts. *Journal of Social Work, 18*(4), 410–430. https://doi.org/10.1177/1468017316654341

Hays, P. A. (2009). Integrating evidence-based practice, cognitive–behavior therapy, and multicultural therapy: Ten steps for culturally competent practice. *Professional Psychology: Research and Practice, 40,* 354–360.

Hays, P. A. (2022). *Addressing cultural complexities in counseling and clinical practice: An intersectional approach* (4th ed.). American Psychological Association.

Iwamasa, G. Y., & Hays, P. A. (Eds.). (2019). *Culturally responsive cognitive behavior therapy: Practice and supervision* (2nd ed.). American Psychological Association. https://doi.org/10.1037/0000119-000

La Roche, M. J. (2021). Changing multicultural guidelines: Clinical and research implications for evidence-based psychotherapies. *Professional Psychology: Research and Practice, 52*(2), 111–120. https://doi-org.ezproxy.lib.utah.edu/10.1037/pro0000347

Pinder-Amaker, S., & Wadsworth, L. (2022). *Did that just happen?! Beyond "diversity"—creating sustainable and inclusive organizations.* Beacon Press.

Sinacore, A. L., Ginsberg, F., & Kassan, A. (2013). Feminist, multicultural, and social justice pedagogies in counseling psychology. In C. Z. Enns & E. N. Williams (Eds.),

*The Oxford handbook of feminist multicultural counseling psychology* (pp. 413–431). Oxford University Press.

Smith, T. B., & Trimble, J. E. (2016). *Foundations of multicultural psychology: Research to inform effective practice*. American Psychological Association. https://doi.org/10.1037/14733-000

Soto, A., Smith, T. B., Griner, D., Rodríguez, M. D., & Bernal, G. (2019). Cultural adaptations and multicultural competence. In J. C. Norcross & B. E. Wampold (Eds.), *Psychotherapy relationships that work: Evidence-based therapist responsiveness* (3rd ed., Vol. 2, pp. 86–132). Oxford University Press. https://doi.org/10.1093/med-psych/9780190843960.003.0004

Sue, D. W., Sue, D., Neville, H. A., & Smith, L. (2022). *Counseling the culturally diverse: Theory and practice* (9th ed.). John Wiley & Sons.

Togans, L., Robinson, L., & Meredith, K. (2014). *Microaggression activity*. In M. Kite (Ed.), *Breaking the prejudice habit*. Ball State University, breakingprejudice.org

Vasquez, M. J. T., & Johnson, J. D. (2022). *Multicultural therapy: A practice imperative*. American Psychological Association. https://doi.org/10.1037/0000279-000

Zimmerman, J., Barnett, J. E., & Campbell, L. F. (Eds.). (2020). *Bringing psychotherapy to the underserved: Challenges and strategies*. Oxford University Press.

## Key Publications for Specific Identity Markers

American Psychological Association. (2019). APA guidelines on race and ethnicity in psychology: Promoting responsiveness and equity. https://www.apa.org/about/policy/guidelines-race-ethnicity.pdf

Carvalho, S. A., Castilho, P., Seabra, D., Salvador, C., Rijo, D., & Carona, C. (2022). Critical issues in cognitive behavioural therapy (CBT) with gender and sexual minorities (GSMs). *The Cognitive Behaviour Therapist*, *15*, E3. https://doi.org/10.1017/S1754470X21000398

Gone, J. P. (2021). Decolonization as methodological innovation in counseling psychology: Method, power, and process in reclaiming American Indian therapeutic traditions. *Journal of Counseling Psychology*, *68*(3), 259–270. https://doi-org.ezproxy.lib.utah.edu/10.1037/cou0000500

Goodman, L. A., Smyth, K. F., & Banyard, V. (2010). Beyond the 50-minute hour: Increasing control, choice, and connections in the lives of low-income women. *American Journal of Orthopsychiatry*, *80*(1), 3. https://doi.org/10.1111/j.1939-0025.2010.01002.x

Hope, D. A., Holt, N. R., Woodruff, N., Mocarski, R., Meyer, H. M., Puckett, J. A., . . . Butler, S. (2022). Bridging the gap between practice guidelines and the therapy room: Community-derived adaptations for psychological services with transgender and gender diverse adults in the Central United States. *Professional Psychology: Research and Practice*, *53*(4), 351–361. https://doi.org/10.1037/pro0000448.

Olkin, R. (2012). Disability: A primer for therapists. In E. M. Altmaier & J.-I. C. Hansen (Eds.), *The Oxford handbook of counseling psychology* (pp. 460–479). Oxford University Press.

Oshin, L. A., Ching, T. H. W., & West, L. M. (2019). Supervising therapist trainees of color. In M. T. Williams, D. C. Rosen, & J. W. Kanter (Eds.), *Eliminating race-based mental health disparities: Promoting equity and culturally responsive care across settings.* (pp. 187–201). Context Press/New Harbinger Publications.

Rosmarin, D. H. (2018). *Spirituality & cognitive behavior therapy: A guide for clinicians.* Guilford Press.

Zane, N., Bernal, G., & Leong, F. (Eds.). (2016). *Evidence-based psychological practice with ethnic minorities: Culturally informed research and clinical strategies.* American Psychological Press. https://doi.org/10.1037/14940-000

## Guideline 4: Local and Regional Cultural Consultation Resources Referenced in Table 4.1

National Alliance for Hispanic Health: https://www.healthyamericas.org
Indian Health Service (INS): https://www.ihs.gov/newsroom/factsheets/behavioralhealth/
Human Rights Campaign (HRC):
    https://www.hrc.org/resources/mental-health-resources-in-the-lgbtq-community
National Deaf Center (NDC): https://www.nationaldeafcenter.org/resources
Rural Health Information Hub: https://www.ruralhealthinfo.org/topics/mental-health
Mental Health America: https://www.mhanational.org/programs
NAMI various community pages:
    https://www.nami.org/Your-Journey/Identity-and-Cultural-Dimensions/
SAMHSA Faith-Based and Community Initiatives:
    https://www.samhsa.gov/faith-based-initiatives

## Guideline 6: Repositories for Understanding Microaggressions

Ball State University discrimination and microaggression reflections:
    www.breakingprejudice.org
More on implicit biases and microaggressions:
    https://www.edutopia.org/article/look-implicit-bias-and-microaggressions

Abbott, D. M., Pelc, N., & Mercier, C. (2019). Cultural humility and the teaching of psychology. *Scholarship of Teaching and Learning in Psychology, 5*(2), 169–181. https://doi-org/10.1037/stl0000144

Ali, A., & Sichel, C. E. (2020). Radicalizing advocacy in service settings: Using structural competency to address tensions between social action and psychological practice. *Psychological Services, 17*(S1), 22–29. https://doi.org/10.1037/ser0000382

American Psychiatric Association. (2013). *Diagnostic and statistical manual of mental disorders* (5th ed.). APA.

American Psychological Association. (2017). *Multicultural guidelines: An ecological approach to context, identity and intersectionality*. APA. http://www.apa.org/about/policy/multicultural-guidelines.pdf.

American Psychological Association. (2019). *APA guidelines on race and ethnicity in psychology: Promoting responsiveness and equity*. APA. http://www.apa.org/about/policy/race-and-ethnicity-in-psychology.pdf

APA Presidential Task Force on Evidence-Based Practice. (2006). Evidence-based practice in psychology. *American Psychologist, 61*, 271–285. https://doi: 10.1037/0003-066X.61.4.271

Asnaani, A., Charlery White, S. R., & Phillip, T.-M. (2020). Mobilizing mental health training efforts to align with advocacy for disenfranchised groups in global contexts: Trauma-related training in the Caribbean as an example. *The Behavior Therapist, 43*(7), 254–260.

Asnaani, A., & Foa, E. B. (2015). Expanding the lens of evidence-based practice in psychotherapy to include a Common Factors perspective: Comment on Laska, Gurman, & Wampold. *Psychotherapy, 51*(4), 487–490.

Asnaani, A., & Hofmann, S. G. (2012). Collaboration in culturally responsive therapy: Establishing a strong therapeutic alliance across cultural lines. *Journal of Clinical Psychology: In Session, 68*(2), 187–197.

Asnaani, A., Majeed, I. M., Kaur, K., & Gutierrez Chavez, M. (2022). Diversity and clinical perspectives in psychology. In G. Asmundson (Ed.), *Comprehensive clinical psychology* (2nd ed., pp. 202–224). Elsevier. https://doi.org/10.1016/B978-0-12-818697-8.00081-9

Asnaani, A., Sanchez-Birkhead, A., Kaur, K., Mukundente, V., Napia, E., Tavake-Pasi, F., . . . Crowell, S. (2022). Utilizing community partnerships to devise a framework for cultural adaptations to evidence-based mental health practice in diverse communities. *Cognitive and Behavioral Practice.* https://doi.org/10.1016/j.cbpra.2022.06.006

Barr, N., Davis, J. P., Diguiseppi, G., Keeling, M., & Castro, C. (2022). Direct and indirect effects of mindfulness, PTSD, and depression on self-stigma of mental illness in OEF/OIF veterans. *Psychological Trauma: Theory, Research, Practice, and Policy, 14*(6), 1026–1034. https://doi.org/10.1037/tra0000535

Bernal, G., Jiménez-Chafey, M. I., & Domenech Rodríguez, M. M. (2009). Cultural adaptation of treatments: A resource for considering culture in evidence-based practice. *Professional Psychology: Research and Practice, 40*(4), 361–368. https://doi.org/10.1037/a0016401

Breland-Noble, A. M., Wong, M. J., Childers, T., Hankerson, S., & Sotomayor, J. (2015). Spirituality and religious coping in African-American youth with depressive illness. *Mental Health, Religion & Culture, 18*(5), 330–341. https://doi.org/10.1080/13674 676.2015.1056120

Burcusa, S. L., & Iacono, W. G. (2007). Risk for recurrence in depression. *Clinical Psychology Review, 27*(8), 959–985. https://doi.org/10.1016/j.cpr.2007.02.005

Carter, R. T., Lau, M. Y., Johnson, V., & Kirkinis, K. (2017). Racial discrimination and health outcomes among racial/ethnic minorities: A meta-analytic review. *Journal of Multicultural Counseling and Development, 45*(4), 232–259.

Carvalho, S. A., Castilho, P., Seabra, D., Salvador, C., Rijo, D., & Carona, C. (2022). Critical issues in cognitive behavioural therapy (CBT) with gender and sexual minorities (GSMs). *The Cognitive Behaviour Therapist, 15,* E3. doi:10.1017/S1754470X21000398

Chandra, R. M., Arora, L., Mehta, U. M., Asnaani, A., & Radhakrishnan, R. (2016). Asian Indians in America: The influence of values and culture on mental health. *Asian Journal of Psychiatry, 22,* 202–209.

Chou, T., Asnaani, A., & Hofmann, S. G. (2012). Perception of racial discrimination and psychopathology across three US ethnic minority groups. *Cultural Diversity and Ethnic Minority Psychology, 18*(1), 74–81. https://doi.org/10.1037/a0025432

Chung, H., & Lu, F. (1996). Ethnocultural factors in the development of an Asian American psychiatrist. *Cultural Diversity and Mental Health, 2,* 99–106.

Commission on Accreditation. (2020, January 1). *Enticing new faces to the field.* American Psychological Association. https://www.apa.org/monitor/ 2020/01/cover-trends-new-faces

Constantine, M. G., & Sue, D. W. (2007). Perceptions of racial microaggressions among Black supervisees in cross-racial dyads. *Journal of Counseling Psychology, 54,* 142–153. https://doi.org/10.1037/0022- 0167.54.2.142

Coronado, S. F., & Peake, T. H. (1992). Culturally sensible therapy: Sensitive principles. *Journal of College Student Psychotherapy, 7,* 63–72.

Craske, M. G., & Barlow, D. H. (2007). *Mastery of your anxiety and panic: Therapist guide* (4th ed.). Oxford University Press.

Cross, T. (2003). Culture as a resource for mental health. *Cultural Diversity and Ethnic Minority Psychology, 9,* 354–359.

Cross, W. E., Jr. (1995). The psychology of Nigrescence: Revising the cross model. In J. G. Ponterotto, J. M. Casas, L. A. Suzuki, & C. M. Alexander (Eds.), *Handbook of multicultural counseling* (pp. 93–122). Sage.

Curcio, C., & Corboy, D. (2020). Stigma and anxiety disorders: A systematic review. *Stigma and Health, 5*(2), 125–137. https://doi.org/10.1037/sah0000183

Danso, R. (2018). Cultural competence and cultural humility: A critical reflection on key cultural diversity concepts. *Journal of Social Work, 18*(4), 410–430. https://doi-org/10.1177/1468017316654341

Davis, D. E., DeBlaere, C., Owen, J., Hook, J. N., Rivera, D. P., Choe, E., . . . Placeres, V. (2018). The multicultural orientation framework: A narrative review. *Psychotherapy, 55*(1), 89–100. https://doi-org/10.1037/pst0000160.supp (Supplemental)

Derr, A. S. (2016). Mental health service use among immigrants in the United States: A systematic review. *Psychiatric Services, 67*(3), 265–274. https://doi.org/10.1176/appi.ps.201500004

Dickerson, D. L., Brown, R. A., Johnson, C. L., Schweigman, K., & D'Amico, E. J. (2016). Integrating motivational interviewing and traditional practices to address alcohol and drug use among urban American Indian/Alaska Native youth. *Journal of Substance Abuse Treatment, 65*, 26–35. https://doi.org/10.1016/j.jsat.2015.06.023

Duan, C. (2020). Serving the underserved: Delivering culturally appropriate service to racial/ethnic minorities. In J. Zimmerman, J. Barnett, & L. Campbell (Eds.), *Bringing psychotherapy to the underserved: Challenges and strategies* (pp. 69–97). Oxford University Press.

Eghaneyan, B. H., & Murphy, E. R. (2020). Measuring mental illness stigma among Hispanics: A systematic review. *Stigma and Health, 5*(3), 351–363. https://doi.org/10.1037/sah0000207

Foa, E. B., Hembree, E. A., Rothbaum, B. O., & Rauch, S. (2019). *Prolonged exposure therapy for PTSD emotional processing of traumatic experiences: Therapist guide.* Oxford University Press.

Foa, E. B., Yadin, E., & Lichner, T. K. (2012). *Exposure and response (ritual) prevention for obsessive-compulsive disorder: Therapist guide* (2nd ed.). Oxford University Press.

Foronda, C., Baptiste, D.-L., Reinholdt, M. M., & Ousman, K. (2016). Cultural humility: A concept analysis. *Journal of Transcultural Nursing, 27*(3), 210–217. https://doi-org/10.1177/1043659615592677

Furukawa, E., & Hunt, D. J. (2011). Therapy with refugees and other immigrants experiencing shame: A multicultural perspective. In R. L. Dearing & J. P. Tangney (Eds.), *Shame in the therapy hour* (pp. 195–215). American Psychological Association.

Gauthier, G., Mucha, L., Shi, S., & Guerin, A. (2019). Economic burden of relapse/recurrence in patients with major depressive disorder. *Journal of Drug Assessment, 8*(1), 97–103. https://doi.org/10.1080/21556660.2019.1612410

Gierk, B., Löwe, B., Murray, A. M., & Kohlmann, S. (2018). Assessment of perceived mental health-related stigma: The Stigma-9 Questionnaire (STIG-9). *Psychiatry Research, 270*, 822–830. https://doi-org/10.1016/j.psychres.2018.10.026

Gilmore, B., & McAuliffe, E. (2013). Effectiveness of community health workers delivering preventive interventions for maternal and child health in low- and middle-income countries: A systematic review. *BMC Public Health, 13*, 847. https://doi:10.1186/1471-2458-13-847

Gómez, J. M. (2020). Trainee perspectives on relational cultural therapy and cultural competency in supervision of trauma cases. *Journal of Psychotherapy Integration*, *30*(1), 60–66. https://doi-org.ezproxy.lib.utah.edu/10.1037/int0000154

Gone, J. P. (2021). Decolonization as methodological innovation in counseling psychology: Method, power, and process in reclaiming American Indian therapeutic traditions. *Journal of Counseling Psychology*, *68*(3), 259–270. https://doi.org/10.1037/cou0000500

Goodman, L. A., Smyth, K. F., & Banyard, V. (2010). Beyond the 50-minute hour: Increasing control, choice, and connections in the lives of low-income women. *American Journal of Orthopsychiatry*, *80*(1), 3. https://doi.org/10.1111/j.1939-0025.2010.01002.x

Greene-Moton, E., & Minkler, M. (2020). Cultural competence or cultural humility? Moving beyond the debate. *Health Promotion Practice*, *21*(1), 142–145. https://doi-org/10.1177/1524839919884912

Gregus, S. J., Stevens, K. T., Seivert, N. P., Tucker, R. P., & Callahan, J. L. (2020). Student perceptions of multicultural training and program climate in Clinical Psychology Doctoral Programs. *Training and Education in Professional Psychology*, *14*(4), 293–307. https://doi.org/10.1037/tep0000289

Griner, D., & Smith, T. B. (2006). Culturally adapted mental health intervention: A meta-analytic review. *Psychotherapy: Theory, Research, Practice, Training*, *43*(4), 531–548. https://doi.org/10.1037/0033-3204.43.4.531

Groen, S. P. N., Richters, A., Laban, C. J., & Devillé, W. L. J. M. (2017). Implementation of the Cultural Formulation through a newly developed Brief Cultural Interview: Pilot data from the Netherlands. *Transcultural Psychiatry*, *54*(1), 3–22. https://doi-org/10.1177/1363461516678342

Gutierrez Chavez, M., Kaur, K., Baucom, K. J. W., Sanchez-Birkhead, A., Sunada, G., Mukundente, V., . . . Asnaani, A. (2022). Developing equitable interventions for ethnically diverse populations: Mental health and co-occurring physical health concerns in the context of the COVID-19 pandemic. *Translational Behavioral Medicine*, *12*(9), 919–926. doi:10.1093/tbm/ibac033. PMID: 36205469; PMCID: PMC9758505.

Hahm, S., Muehlan, H., Stolzenburg, S., Tomczyk, S., Schmidt, S., & Schomerus, G. (2020). How stigma interferes with symptom awareness: Discrepancy between objective and subjective cognitive performance in currently untreated persons with mental health problems. *Stigma and Health*, *5*(2), 146–157. https://doi.org/10.1037/sah0000184

Hair, H. (2015). Supervision conversations about social justice and social work practice. *Journal of Social Work*, *15*(4), 349–370. https://doi:10.1177/1468017314539082

Hall, W. J., Chapman, M. V., Lee, K. M., Merino, Y. M., Thomas, T. W., Payne, B. K., . . . Coyne-Beasley, T. (2015). Implicit racial/ethnic bias among health care professionals and its influence on health care outcomes: A systematic review. *American Journal of Public Health*, *105*(12), e60–e76. https://doi-org.ezproxy.lib.utah.edu/10.2105/AJPH.2015.302903

Halpert, S. C., & Pfaller, J. (2001). Sexual orientation and supervision: Theory and practice. *Journal of Gay & Lesbian Social Services: Issues in Practice, Policy & Research*, *13*(3), 23–40. https://doi-org.ezproxy.lib.utah.edu/10.1300/J041v13n03_02

Hays, P. A. (2009). Integrating evidence-based practice, cognitive–behavior therapy, and multicultural therapy: Ten steps for culturally competent practice. *Professional Psychology: Research and Practice*, *40*, 354–360.

Hays, P. A. (2022). *Addressing cultural complexities in counseling and clinical practice: An intersectional approach* (4th ed.). American Psychological Association.

Helms, J. E. (1995). An update of Helms's White and people of color racial identity models. In J. G. Ponterotto, J. M. Casas, L. A. Suzuki, & D. M. Alexander (Eds.), *Handbook of multicultural counseling* (pp. 181–198). Sage.

Hernández, P., & McDowell, T. (2010). Intersectionality, power, and relational safety in context: Key concepts in clinical supervision. *Training and Education in Professional Psychology*, 4(1), 29–35. https://doi-org/10.1037/a0017064

Hollon, S. D., DeRubeis, R. J., Shelton, R. C., Amsterdam, J. D., Salomon, R. M., O'Reardon, J. P., . . . Gallop, R. (2005). Prevention of relapse following cognitive therapy vs medications in moderate to severe depression. *Archives of General Psychiatry*, 62(4), 417–422. https://doi-org/10.1001/archpsyc.62.4.417

Hook, J. N., Davis, D. E., Owen, J., Worthington, E. L., & Utsey, S. O. (2013). Cultural humility: Measuring openness to culturally diverse clients. *Journal of Counseling Psychology*, 60(3), 353–366. https://doi.org/10.1037/a0032595

Hope, D. A., Holt, N. R., Woodruff, N., Mocarski, R., Meyer, H., Puckett, J. A., . . . Butler, S. (2022). Bridging the gap between practice guidelines and the therapy room: Community-derived adaptations for psychological services with transgender and gender diverse adults in the Central United States. *Professional Psychology: Research and Practice*, 53(4), 351–361. https://doi.org/10.1037/pro 0000448.

Horne, S. G., Maroney, M. R., Nel, J. A., Chaparro, R. A., & Manalastas, E. J. (2019). Emergence of a transnational LGBTI psychology: Commonalities and challenges in advocacy and activism. *American Psychologist*, 74(8), 967–986. https://doi.org/10.1037/amp0000561

Jackson, J. S., & Williams, D. (2002). *Detroit area study, 1995: Social influence on health: Stress, racism, and health protective resources.* Inter-university Consortium for Political and Social Research. https://doi.org/10.3886/ICPSR03272.v1

Jernigan, M. M., Green, C. E., Helms, J. E., Perez-Gualdron, L., & Henze, K. (2010). An examination of people of color supervision dyads: Racial identity matters as much as race. *Training and Education in Professional Psychology*, 4(1), 62–73. https://doi-org/10.1037/a0018110

Kaur, K., Gutierrez Chavez, M., Tacana, T., Sanchez-Birkhead, A., Mukundente, V., Napia, E. E., . . . Asnaani, A. (2022). Applying best practices for health disparities work to create a treatment adaptation framework for culturally diverse communities: A mixed-methods approach. *Journal of Consulting and Clinical Psychology*, 90(10), 734–746. https://doi.org/10.1037/ccp0000742

Kelly, J. F., & Greene, B. (2010). Diversity within African American, female therapists: Variability in clients' expectations and assumptions about the therapist. *Psychotherapy: Theory, Research, Practice, Training*, 47(2), 186–197. https://doi-org/10.1037/a0019759

Kelly, S. (2006). Cognitive-behavioral therapy with African Americans. In P. A. Hays & G. Y. Iwamasa (Eds.), *Culturally responsive cognitive-behavioral therapy: Assessment, practice, and supervision* (pp. 97–116). American Psychological Association.

Knowles, E. D., Lowery, B. S., Chow, R. M., & Unzueta, M. M. (2014). Deny, distance, or dismantle? How white Americans manage a privileged identity. *Perspectives on Psychological Science*, 9(6), 594–609. https://doi.org/10.1177/1745691614554658

La Roche, M. J. (2021). Changing multicultural guidelines: Clinical and research implications for evidence-based psychotherapies. *Professional Psychology: Research and Practice*, *52*(2), 111–120. https://doi-org.ezproxy.lib.utah.edu/10.1037/pro 0000347

Lau, A. S., Chang, D. F., & Okazaki, S. (2010). Methodological challenges in treatment outcome research with ethnic minorities. *Cultural Diversity and Ethnic Minority Psychology*, *16*, 573–580. https://dx.doi.org/10.1037%2Fa0021371

Lee, A., & Khawaja, N. G. (2013). Multicultural training experiences as predictors of psychology students' cultural competence. *Australian Psychologist*, *48*(3), 209–216. https://doi-org/10.1111/j.1742-9544.2011.00063.x

Lee, A. T., & Haskins, N. H. (2022). Toward a culturally humble practice: Critical consciousness as an antecedent. *Journal of Counseling & Development*, *100*(1), 104–112. https://doi.org/10.1002/jcad.12403

Lee, E., Tsang, A. K. T., Bogo, M., Johnstone, M., & Herschman, J. (2018). Enactments of racial microaggression in everyday therapeutic encounters. *Smith College Studies in Social Work*, *88*(3), 211–236. https://doi-org/10.1080/00377317.2018.1476646

Levy, H. C., Stevens, K. T., & Tolin, D. F. (2022). Research review: A meta-analysis of relapse rates in cognitive behavioral therapy for anxiety and related disorders in youth. *Journal of Child Psychology and Psychiatry*, *63*(3), 252–260. https://doi/org/ 10.1111/jcpp.13486

Lipscomb, A. E., & Ashley, W. (2017). Colorful disclosures: Identifying identity-based differences and enhancing critical consciousness in supervision. *Smith College Studies in Social Work*, *87*(2–3), 220–237. https://doi-org.ezproxy.lib.utah.edu/ 10.1080/00377317.2017.1324098

Mackenzie, C. S., Heath, P. J., Vogel, D. L., & Chekay, R. (2019). Age differences in public stigma, self-stigma, and attitudes toward seeking help: A moderated mediation model. *Journal of Clinical Psychology*, *75*(12), 2259–2272. https://doi.org/10.1002/ jclp.22845

Mangione, L., Borden, K. A., Nadkarni, L., Evarts, K., & Hyde, K. (2018). Mentoring in clinical psychology programs: Broadening and deepening. *Training and Education in Professional Psychology*, *12*(1), 4. https://psycnet.apa.org/doi/10.1037/tep0000167

Marshal, M. P., Dietz, L. J., Friedman, M. S., Stall, R., Smith, H. A., McGinley, J., . . . Brent, D. A. (2011). Suicidality and depression disparities between sexual minority and heterosexual youth: A meta-analytic review. *Journal of Adolescent Health*, *49*(2), 115–123. https://doi.org/10.1016/j.jadohealth.2011.02.005

Martell, C. R., Dimidjian, S., & Herman-Dunn, R. (2010). *Behavioral activation for depression: A clinician's guide*. Guilford Press.

Maxie, A. C., & Arnold, D. H. (2006). Do therapists address ethnic and racial differences in cross-cultural psychotherapy? *Psychotherapy: Theory, Research, Practice, Training*, *43*, 85–98.

Meyer, I. H. (2003). Prejudice, social stress, and mental health in lesbian, gay, and bisexual populations: Conceptual issues and research evidence. *Psychological Bulletin*, *129*(5), 674. https://dx.doi.org/10.1037%2F0033-2909.129.5.674

Murphy-Shigematsu, S. (2010). Microaggressions by supervisors of color. *Training and Education in Professional Psychology*, *4*(1), 16–18. https://doi-org/10.1037/a0017472

Nadal, K. L., Davidoff, K. C., Davis, L. S., Wong, Y., Marshall, D., & McKenzie, V. (2015). A qualitative approach to intersectional microaggressions: Understanding influences of race, ethnicity, gender, sexuality, and religion. *Qualitative Psychology*, *2*(2), 146–163. https://psycnet.apa.org/doi/10.1037/qup0000026

Olkin, R. (2012). Disability: A primer for therapists. In E. M. Altmaier & J.-I. C. Hansen (Eds.), *The Oxford handbook of counseling psychology* (pp. 460–479). Oxford University Press.

Oshin, L. A., Ching, T. H. W., & West, L. M. (2019). Supervising therapist trainees of color. In M. T. Williams, D. C. Rosen, & J. W. Kanter (Eds.), *Eliminating race-based mental health disparities: Promoting equity and culturally responsive care across settings* (pp. 187–201). Context Press/New Harbinger Publications.

Owen, J., Leach, M. M., Wampold, B., & Rodolfa, E. (2010). Client and therapist variability in clients' perceptions of their therapists' multicultural competencies. *Journal of Counseling Psychology*, *58*, 1–9.

Owen, J., Drinane, J. M., Tao, K. W., DasGupta, D. R., Zhang, Y. S. D., & Adelson, J. (2018). An experimental test of microaggression detection in psychotherapy: Therapist multicultural orientation. *Professional Psychology: Research and Practice*, *49*(1), 9–21. https://doi-org/10.1037/pro0000152

Owen, J., Tao, K. W., Drinane, J. M., Hook, J., Davis, D. E., & Kune, N. F. (2016). Client perceptions of therapists' multicultural orientation: Cultural (missed) opportunities and cultural humility. *Professional Psychology: Research and Practice*, *47*(1), 30–37. https://doi.org/10.1037/pro0000046

Owen, J., Tao, K. W., Imel, Z. E., Wampold, B. E., & Rodolfa, E. (2014). Addressing racial and ethnic microaggressions in therapy. *Professional Psychology: Research and Practice*, *45*(4), 283–290.

Pfohl, A. H. (2004). The intersection of personal and professional identity: The heterosexual supervisor's role in fostering the development of sexual minority supervisees. *The Clinical Supervisor*, *23*(1), 139–164. https://doi-org/10.1300/J001v23n01_09

Pilkington, N. W., & Cantor, J. M. (1996). Perceptions of heterosexual bias in professional psychology programs: A survey of graduate students. *Professional Psychology: Research and Practice*, *27*(6), 604–612. https://doi-org/10.1037/0735-7028.27.6.604

Pinder-Amaker, S., & Wadsworth, L. (2022). *Did that just happen?! Beyond "diversity—creating sustainable and inclusive organizations.* Beacon Press.

Plaut, V. C. (2010). Diversity science: Why and how difference makes a difference. *Psychological Inquiry*, *21*, 77–99. https://psycnet.apa.org/doi/10.1080/10478401003676501

Plummer, D. L. (1997). A Gestalt approach to culturally responsive mental health treatment. *Gestalt Review*, *1*, 190–204.

Quintana, S. M. (2007). Racial and ethnic identity: Developmental perspectives and research. *Journal of Counseling Psychology*, *54*, 259–270.

Rathod, S., Gega, L., Degnan, A., Pikard, J., Khan, T., Husain, N., . . . Naeem, F. (2018). The current status of culturally adapted mental health interventions: A practice-focused review of meta-analyses. *Neuropsychiatric Disease and Treatment*, *14*, 165–178. https://doi.org/10.2147/NDT.S138430

Rimes, K. A., Ion, D., Wingrove, J., & Carter, B. (2019). Sexual orientation differences in psychological treatment outcomes for depression and anxiety: National cohort study. *Journal of Consulting and Clinical Psychology*, *87*(7), 577–589. https://doi.org/10.1037/ccp0000416.supp(Supplemental)

Roberts, R. E., Phinney, J. S., Masse, L. C., Chen, Y. R., Roberts, C. R., & Romero, A. (1999). The structure of ethnic identity of young adolescents from diverse ethnocultural groups. *Journal of Early Adolescence*, *19*, 301–322. http://dx.doi.org/ 10.1177/ 0272431699019003001

Rodriguez, N., Myers, H. F., Mira, C. B., Flores, T., & Garcia-Hernandez, L. (2002). Development of the Multidimensional Acculturative Stress Inventory for adults of Mexican origin. *Psychological Assessment*, *14*(4), 451–461. https://doi-org/10.1037/ 1040-3590.14.4.451

Roemer, L., & Orsillo, S. M. (2020). Acceptance-based behavioral therapies for generalized anxiety disorder (GAD). In A. L. Gerlach & A. T. Gloster (Eds.), *Generalized anxiety disorder and worrying: A comprehensive handbook for clinicians and researchers* (pp. 245–271). Wiley Blackwell. https://doi.org/10.1002/9781119189909.ch12

Roemer, L., & Orsillo, S. M. (2020). *Acceptance-based behavioral therapy: Treating anxiety and related challenges* (4th ed.). Guilford Press.

Rosmarin, D. H. (2018). *Spirituality & cognitive behavior therapy: A guide for clinicians.* Guilford Press.

Rovitto, T. L. (2022). (Cultural) humility in practice: Engaging first-generation college students. *Journal of College Student Psychotherapy*, *36*(3), 294–309. https://doi.org/ 10.1080/87568225.2020.1819924

Ryder, A. G., Alden, L. E., & Paulhus, D. L. (2000). Is acculturation unidimensional or bidimensional? A head-to-head comparison in the prediction of personality, self-identity, and adjustment. *Journal of Personality and Social Psychology*, *79*(1), 49–65. https://doi.org/10.1037/0022-3514.79.1.49

Sam, D. L., & Berry, J. W. (2010). Acculturation: When individuals and groups of different cultural backgrounds meet. *Perspectives on Psychological Science*, *5*(4), 472–481. https://doi.org/10.1177/1745691610373075

Shea, M., & Yeh, C. J. (2008). Asian American students' cultural values, stigma, and relational self-construal: Correlates of attitudes toward professional help seeking. *Journal of Mental Health Counseling*, *30*, 157–172. https://psycnet.apa.org/doi/ 10.17744/mehc.30.2.g662g5l2r1352198

Shelton, K., & Delgado-Romero, E. (2011). Sexual orientation microaggressions: The experience of lesbian, gay, bisexual, and queer clients in psychotherapy. *Journal of Counseling Psychology*, *58*(2), 210–221.

Sinacore, A. L., Ginsberg, F., & Kassan, A. (2013). Feminist, multicultural, and social justice pedagogies in counseling psychology. In C. Z. Enns & E. N. Williams (Eds.), *The Oxford handbook of feminist multicultural counseling psychology* (pp. 413–431). Oxford University Press.

Singelis, T. M. (1994). The measurement of independent and interdependent self-construals. *Personality and Social Psychology Bulletin*, *20*(5), 580–591. https://doi-org/10.1177/0146167294205014

Sirin, S. R., Ryce, P., Gupta, T., & Rogers-Sirin, L. (2013). The role of acculturative stress on mental health symptoms for immigrant adolescents: A longitudinal investigation. *Developmental Psychology*, *49*(4), 736–748. https://psycnet.apa.org/doi/ 10.1037/a0028398

Skitka, L. J., & Crosby, F. J. (2003). Trends in the social psychological study of justice. *Personality and Social Psychology Review*, *7*(4), 282–285. https://doi.org/10.1207/ S15327957PSPR0704_01

Smith, T. B., & Trimble, J. E. (2016). *Foundations of multicultural psychology: Research to inform effective practice*. American Psychological Association. https://doi.org/10.1037/14733-000

Soto, A., Smith, T. B., Griner, D., Rodríguez, M. D., & Bernal, G. (2019). Cultural adaptations and multicultural competence. In J. C. Norcross & B. E. Wampold (Eds.), Psychotherapy relationships that work: Evidence-based therapist responsiveness (3rd ed., Vol. 2, pp. 86–132). Oxford University Press. https://doi-org.ezproxy.lib.utah.edu/10.1093/med-psych/9780190843960.003.0004Sue, D. W., Alsaidi, S., Awad, M. N., Glaeser, E., Calle, C. Z., & Mendez, N. (2019). Disarming racial microaggressions: Microintervention strategies for targets, White allies, and bystanders. *American Psychologist, 74*(1), 128–142. https://doi-org/10.1037/amp0000296

Sue, D. W., Capodilupo, C. M., Torino, G. C., Bucceri, J. M., Holder, A. M. B., Nadal, K. L., & Esquilin, M. (2007). Racial microaggressions in everyday life: Implications for clinical practice. *American Psychologist, 62*, 271–286.

Sue, D. W., & Sue, D. (2008). Racial/cultural identity development in People of Color. In D. W. Sue & D. Sue (Eds.), *Counseling the culturally diverse: Theory and practice* (pp. 233–258). John Wiley & Sons.

Sue, D. W., Sue, D., Neville, H. A., & Smith, L. (2022). *Counseling the culturally diverse: Theory and practice* (9th ed.). John Wiley & Sons.

Sue, S. (1998). In search of cultural competence in psychotherapy and counseling. *American Psychologist, 53*, 440–448. https://psycnet.apa.org/doi/10.1037/0003-066X.53.4.440

Sue, S., & Zane, N. (2009). The role of culture and cultural techniques in psychotherapy: A critique and reformulation. *Asian American Journal of Psychology, 1*, 3–14.

Taber, B. J., Leibert, T. W., & Agaskar, V. R. (2011). Relationships among client-therapist personality congruence, working alliance, and therapeutic outcome. *Psychotherapy (Chic), 48*(4), 376–380.

Tao, K. W., Owen, J., Pace, B. T., & Imel, Z. E. (2015). A meta-analysis of multicultural competencies and psychotherapy process and outcome. *Journal of Counseling Psychology, 62*(3), 337–350.

Taylor, R. E., & Kuo, B. C. H. (2019). Black American psychological help-seeking intention: An integrated literature review with recommendations for clinical practice. *Journal of Psychotherapy Integration, 29*(4), 325–337. https://doi-org/10.1037/int0000131

Togans, L., Robinson, L., & Meredith, K. (2014). Microaggression activity. In M. Kite (Ed.), *Breaking the prejudice habit*. Ball State University, breakingprejudice.org.

Triandis, H. C., & Gelfland, M. J. (1998). Converging measurement of horizontal and vertical individualism and collectivism. *Journal of Personality and Social Psychology, 74*, 118–128.

Umaña-Taylor, A. J., Yazedjian, A., & Bámaca-Gómez, M. Y. (2004). Developing the Ethnic Identity Scale using Eriksonian and social identity perspectives. *Identity: An International Journal of Theory and Research, 4*, 9–38.

Vasquez, M. J. T. (2007). Cultural difference and the therapeutic alliance: An evidence-based analysis. *American Psychologist, 62*, 878–885.

Vasquez, M. J. T., & Johnson, J. D. (2022). Summary. In M. J. T. Vasquez & J. D. Johnson (Eds.), *Multicultural therapy: A practice imperative* (pp. 153–164). American Psychological Association. https://doi.org/10.1037/0000279-007

Vogel, D. L., Wade, N. G., & Haake, S. (2006). Measuring the self-stigma associated with seeking psychological help. *Journal of Counseling Psychology*, *53*(3), 325–337.https://doi.org/10.1037/0022-0167.53.3.325

Williams, D. R., Yu, Y., Jackson, J. S., & Anderson, N. B. (1997). Racial differences in physical and mental health: Socio-economic status, stress and discrimination. *Journal of Health Psychology*, *2*, 335–351.

Williams, M. T., Metzger, I. W., Leins, C., & DeLapp, C. (2018). Assessing racial trauma within a DSM–5 framework: The UConn Racial/Ethnic Stress & Trauma Survey. *Practice Innovations*, *3*(4), 242–260. https://doi-org/10.1037/pri0000076.supp (Supplemental)

Witkiewitz, K. A., & Marlatt, G. A. (Eds.). (2007). *Therapist's guide to evidence-based relapse prevention*. Elsevier Academic Press.

World Health Organization. (2017). *Global strategy and action plan on ageing and health*. WHO. License: CC BY-NC-SA 3.0 IGO.

Zane, N., Bernal, G., & Leong, F. (Eds.). (2016). *Evidence-based psychological practice with ethnic minorities: Culturally informed research and clinical strategies*. American Psychological Press. https://doi.org/10.1037/ 14940-000

Zhang, C.-Q., Leeming, E., Smith, P., Chung, P.-K., Hagger, M. S., & Hayes, S. C. (2018). Acceptance and commitment therapy for health behavior change: A contextually-driven approach. *Frontiers in Psychology*, *8*. https://doi.org/10.3389/fpsyg.2017.02350